# Flourishing
## WITH
# FIBROMYALGIA

YOUR NATURAL GUIDE TO TAKING BACK THE
LIFE FIBROMYALGIA STOLE FROM YOU

DR. MELYSSA HOITINK, ND

# Download the Flourishing with Fibromyalgia Action Guide FREE!

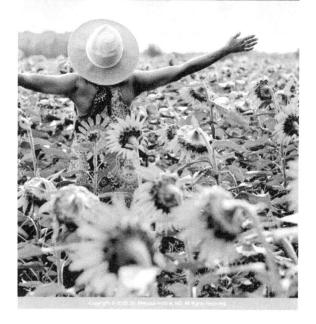

## READ THIS FIRST

To say thanks for buying my book, I would like to give you the Flourishing with Fibromyalgia Action Guide 100% FREE!

### TO DOWNLOAD GO TO:
https://resources.flourishingwithfibromyalgia.com/fibromyalgia-action-guide

# Dedication

This book is dedicated to the three most influential women in my life, my wonderful mom, Aunt Karen, and Aunt Lynda. None of this would have been possible without your support and encouragement.

# TABLE OF CONTENTS

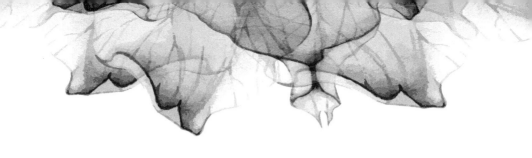

# SECTION 1

## Understanding Fibromyalgia

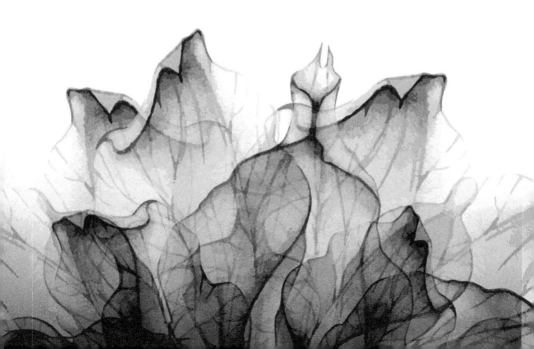

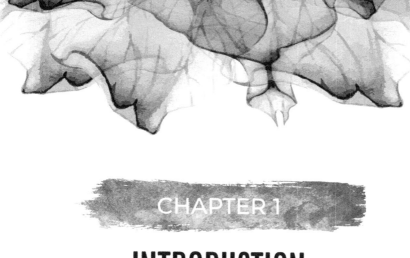

# CHAPTER 1

# INTRODUCTION

## WHO IS THIS BOOK FOR?

Do you suffer from a wide variety of symptoms, but medical professionals have yet to tell you what is causing them? Or maybe you've heard of fibromyalgia before, or someone has mentioned to you that they thought you had it? Fibromyalgia is a complex condition, and medicine is still in the process of explaining what causes it, how to diagnose it, and how to treat it effectively. I've written this book to kick-start your journey to living the life you've always dreamed of, without the symptoms of fibromyalgia getting in your way.

Fibromyalgia most often affects women who are the caretakers of their families, the go-to people at work who always get the job done, those who everyone expects will be the boss one day (or maybe already are). Fibromyalgia sufferers are the people who are the foundation of the group around them. This condition affects women who have big dreams and goals for what they want their lives to look like.

If fibromyalgia has taken control of your body, your brain, and your life, it is limiting you from reaching your true potential. That stops right here in this book. This book is written for women, just like you, who have big goals and dreams. Women who want to live symptom-free and achieve those dreams. This book contains information both for women who are not sure if they have fibromyalgia and women who have been already diagnosed, either recently or years ago. If you are suffering from symptoms of fibromyalgia, this book contains strategies and options that can get you back to the life you've always dreamed of, despite your diagnosis.

## WHO IS THIS BOOK NOT FOR?

This book is packed with strategies to address fibromyalgia using natural therapies and lifestyle and dietary changes. This book is not for people looking for information on pharmaceutical treatment options for fibromyalgia. While pharmaceutical medication can be immensely helpful in the treatment of fibromyalgia and is something that you should explore in order to be fully informed of your treatment options, it is not a topic discussed in detail in this book. Please speak with your medical doctor or pharmacist to learn more about the pharmaceutical options for treating fibromyalgia.

This book is also not intended for people who do not wish to get better. If you are fine with the symptoms you're experiencing, no matter how debilitating, or if you believe there is absolutely no hope for living well with fibromyalgia, your time will be better spent elsewhere. This book is for people who believe they can get better and who are ready and willing to take the necessary steps to do so.

## WHO AM I AND WHY AM I WRITING A BOOK ON FIBROMYALGIA?

I'm Dr. Melyssa, a naturopathic doctor in Barrie, Ontario, Canada. I have never been diagnosed with fibromyalgia, so why do I care enough to write a book on the topic? My experience in no way compares to the severity of living with fibromyalgia, but I can identify with parts of the experience and how it made me feel. I can see how the experience of women with fibromyalgia in the world and in the medical system could dim their lights and result in the internal belief that they will never get better. I can imagine how it could feel and how it could have limited my potential if it had happened to me on a grander scale and more frequently. I can imagine how discouraging it can feel to have your body not cooperate with your plan for your life.

As a teenager I suffered from severe migraines, debilitating painful periods, and constant back and neck pain. I was sore all over, all the time. I was exhausted from the pain and from trying to pretend that I didn't feel it. From the outside, I appeared to have it all. I got good grades in school, and I helped tutor other students. I was athletic and artistic, winning awards in most sports or extracurricular activities that I tried. I worked a part-time job and still managed to have a full social life. My life at home was a different story. My dad passed away when I was nine years old, after a long battle with brain cancer. Being the quintessential "daddy's girl," I was devastated. My home life became much more unstable. My mom struggled with addiction and the stress of raising four children. My brothers and I were separated and shuffled from home to home, as we tried to maintain a normal teenage life.

5

In high school, I began seeing doctors about the pain, which was preventing me from attending school, playing the sports I loved, going to work, and seeing my friends. In our ten-minute sessions, my doctors prescribed pain-relieving and anti-inflammatory medications and sent me for blood tests and imaging. The tests all came back normal, and the medications didn't take the pain away. I was told that the medications should relieve the pain, and the only way they wouldn't is if I were making it all up. After all, "kids who come from my kind of home life didn't get enough attention." I'd heard this line from teachers, friends' parents, and relatives before. I must be making it up for attention, because normal teenagers didn't experience the pain I did. The underlying message was that I would never get better, and pain medications were my only option, as long as I felt the need to seek attention for my made-up symptoms. The more often I was told this, the closer I came to believing it.

I started university wanting to become a medical doctor. I wanted to help people live a healthy life, and I wanted them to leave my office feeling better than they had ever felt before. I wanted to give people a better experience than I had in my health journey. I quickly came to realize that the medical system we have in North America is not set up to support this type of medicine. Visits are short and we use Band-Aid approaches (medications you take for a lifetime), because that is less expensive in the short term than taking the time to teach people how to eat healthy, live healthy, and fix the root cause of their problems.

Feeling a little lost, I attended a job fair at my university and stumbled across a naturopathic doctor. I had never heard of a naturopathic doctor before, and I was intrigued. A form of medicine that takes the time to really get to know the patient and then uses natural therapies to heal them and prevent future health issues—sign me up! I booked my first appointment with my new naturopathic doctor. My naturopathic doctor worked with me to identify problems in my diet and lifestyle and supported me in making changes. She educated me on the importance of sleep and seeking support for my emotional state. She discussed my body's natural response to stress and how this can manifest as physical symptoms. She recommended supplements to relieve my symptoms, address what was truly causing them, and provide my body with the nutrients necessary to heal. While working with my first naturopathic doctor I became migraine-free, with greatly reduced pain and a higher level of energy. I felt like I could take on the world again! I decided that naturopathic medicine was exactly what I had been looking for, and I started my education to become a naturopathic doctor.

During my schooling to become a naturopathic doctor, I was lucky enough to be selected to work as an intern on a clinical shift focused specifically on caring for people with fibromyalgia and myalgic encephalomyelitis (also known as chronic fatigue syndrome). I did not understand at the time how much I would learn and the impact it would have on my life.

In my time spent on this shift, I realized that the women I was working with were a lot like me. They had big dreams for their careers, their families, and their success. They wanted to make a big impact in the world. They wanted to have it all, and if someone told them they couldn't do it, they worked that much harder to prove them wrong. All was fine and well in their lives, until they began experiencing the symptoms of fibromyalgia. Instead of going on to reach their career goals, raise wonderful children, and discover solutions to the world's big problems, they became nearly bedridden most days because of pain and fatigue. They lost their ability to think clearly and problem solve as they once could. I believe the world has lost some of its biggest change seekers because of fibromyalgia. I find women with fibromyalgia to be incredibly inspiring, engaged in their health journey, and well-educated on their condition. These women do not give up, and they do not let challenges stop them from continuing to try to live a better life.

In my time spent as an intern and in my clinical practice since graduating, I've seen the impact that natural therapies, diet modifications, and lifestyle changes can make for women with fibromyalgia. I've seen kind and generous women who've felt discouraged and hopeless about their health take back control of their lives and become symptom-free. I've seen these women achieve big goals, like getting the promotion they've always wanted, writing a book, starting a family, and helping others who were in their shoes. This can be you. I believe this with all my being, and you should too.

## WHY DOES THIS BOOK MATTER?

This book matters because you deserve the best medical care possible. You deserve to live the life you have always dreamed of and more. You do not have to suffer forever, despite the resounding messages you are bombarded with every day. You deserve to be informed of your options so that you can make the best decisions for yourself. You know your body best, and not every treatment or combination of treatments will work for every person. You are an individual, and you deserve better than cookie-cutter medicine. Not only do you deserve all these things, the world deserves to experience the positive impact you will make by achieving your dreams.

## HOW IS THIS BOOK DIFFERENT FROM ANY OTHER BOOK ON FIBROMYALGIA?

There are several great books on fibromyalgia already in existence (check out the Additional Resources section or download your own copy here: https://resources.flourishingwithfibromyalgia.com/fibromyalgia-resource-guide, if you're interested in others). In reviewing the content of other books and resources, I was struck by how little actionable information is given on key dietary and lifestyle changes and how little information is given on natural therapies. Knowledge is nice and good to have, but how do you actually put any of this into practice to improve your health?

Your journey to living well with fibromyalgia starts right here in this book. Don't forget to grab your copy of the Flourishing With Fibromyalgia Action Guide (https://resources.flourishingwithfibromyalgia.com/fibromyalgia-action-guide) and the Flourishing With Fibromyalgia Resource Guide (https://resources.flourishingwithfibromyalgia.com/fibromyalgia-resource-guide) as your quick reference companion guides to this book.

## DISCLAIMER

This book does not replace the advice of a qualified health care provider. This book is intended to be as thorough as possible, but you are an individual, and your experience is not necessarily the same as others with fibromyalgia. Your health will always include aspects unique to you. For this reason, it is always important to seek medical advice for your specific health condition. Supplements and natural therapies carry risks and the possibility of adverse effects, just like prescription medications. It is also possible for natural therapies to interact with prescription medications. I've included information on when to avoid specific supplements; however, this information is not exhaustive and does not replace the advice of your health care providers. Please always be sure to check with your health care providers to be sure a new treatment option is safe for you.

**Note on Dosing:** I have included information on dosing of natural treatment options based on the available research and my clinical experience; however, some people with fibromyalgia are sensitive to supplements and herbal treatment options. If you are sensitive, your body may not tolerate full doses of any treatment, whether natural or not. If you feel better at a lower dose than what is discussed here, that is perfectly fine. Listen to your body, and don't take a dose that doesn't work for you. It may be helpful to increase doses of new supplements gradually. See the Additional Resources section or grab your free copy here: https://resources.flourishingwithfibromyalgia.com/fibromyalgia-resource-guide for more tips on how to find a dose that works for you.

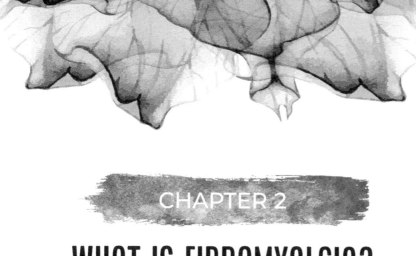

# CHAPTER 2

# WHAT IS FIBROMYALGIA?

## WHO HAS FIBROMYALGIA AND HOW DOES IT DEVELOP?

Fibromyalgia affects approximately 2%–8% of the world's population.[1] It is estimated that 1%–5% of Canadians have fibromyalgia,[2] which equates to approximately 378,000 to 1.8 million Canadians. In the United States, this number is approximately five to ten million adults.[3] These numbers are staggering, yet very few people know what fibromyalgia is.

It is estimated that 75%–90% of people with fibromyalgia are women.[3] It can begin in childhood but is most often diagnosed in adulthood, between the ages of 20 to 50 years.[4] Obtaining a diagnosis of fibromyalgia can be a long and involved process, taking up to five years or more.[5] Many people remain undiagnosed despite meeting all of the criteria.

In my clinical experience and research, I have found that people with fibromyalgia tend to have a similar personality type. This is not to say that personality is a cause of fibromyalgia, but I think it is correlated with how fibromyalgia develops and may be helpful in treatment. The women I meet with fibromyalgia are highly ambitious, always on the run, perfectionist-type people.[6] They are the people you ask when you need something done, and you need it done well. They are very kind, caring, and generous.[6] They have big hearts, big plans for the future, and want to leave the world better than they found it. It is the inherent nature of these women to put others before themselves, even if that is detrimental to their own well-being.[6] I think that this pattern of putting others' needs before one's own contributes to the development of fibromyalgia and makes it more difficult to put your own health first when you are working to get better.

A common theme in the patient histories of people with fibromyalgia is trauma.[7] The experienced trauma can be physical, mental, or emotional. Examples of trauma reported by patients with fibromyalgia may include surgery, motor vehicle accident, whiplash injury, childbirth, infection, other physical injury, abuse (sexual, physical, or emotional), war, natural disasters, childhood traumatic experiences, and stressful life events, such as divorce or the death of a loved one.[7] A history of trauma is not always present in people with fibromyalgia, and you can still be diagnosed with fibromyalgia if you have not experienced a traumatic event.

In my work with women with fibromyalgia, I have often wondered about the connection to intergenerational trauma and the role of repressed trauma in the development of fibromyalgia. Intergenerational trauma is trauma experienced by our ancestors that makes a mark on our DNA and is passed down to later generations. This may contribute to the increased risk of developing fibromyalgia if you have a family member with fibromyalgia. Trauma can become repressed as our body's way of protecting us from particularly painful events. The reason I point out this connection to trauma is that it can give us clues as to where the body is not functioning properly and help uncover the root cause of fibromyalgia.

There is now strong evidence that fibromyalgia has a genetic component.[8–10] If you have a family member with fibromyalgia, you are much more likely to be diagnosed yourself.[1,8] There are also a number of genes that have been linked with the development of fibromyalgia.[8–10] Studies performed on twins suggest that about half of the risk is related to genetics and the other half to environmental factors.[8] This means that even if you have the predisposing genes or a family member with fibromyalgia, you will not necessarily develop it. Genes can be turned on or off by specific events or conditions you are exposed to. Research is ongoing into which genes are implicated, how these genes affect the functioning of the body, and the role played by environmental factors in the development of fibromyalgia.

## WHAT IS PHYSICALLY ABNORMAL IN THE BODY OF SOMEONE WITH FIBROMYALGIA?

You may have heard that your fibromyalgia symptoms are all in your head. This is absolutely not true and is one of the most condescending statements that can be uttered by health care professionals. Research has uncovered a variety of physiological abnormalities in people with fibromyalgia. Anyone who says otherwise has not read the research. If your health care provider says this to you, find a new health care provider.

Research performed on muscle biopsies taken from people with and without fibromyalgia has shown a number of structural, functional, and metabolic differences between these two populations.[11] The structure of muscle tissue in people with fibromyalgia shows a moth-eaten appearance, abnormalities in the appearance of individual muscle fibres, and abnormalities in the cell membranes of muscle cells on biopsy.[11,12] Some degeneration of certain types of muscle fibres also appears to be present compared to healthy controls.[11,12] Blood flow to the muscles appears to be compromised in people with fibromyalgia. Biopsies show a decreased number of capillaries (small blood vessels) and thicker capillary walls within muscle tissue, which may contribute to abnormal oxygen distribution in the muscles of people with fibromyalgia.[11,13] When capillary walls are too thick, gases and metabolites cannot pass through as they normally would. This abnormality in blood flow and oxygen concentration is particularly apparent during exercise, which likely contributes to symptoms of pain, fatigue, and difficulty exercising.[11] Research has shown that people with fibromyalgia use the same amount of energy to perform less work compared to healthy participants.[11] This research supports the observation that people with fibromyalgia have difficulty with tasks requiring muscular endurance.[11]

If you've been reading up on fibromyalgia, it's very likely that you've come across the term *mitochondrial dysfunction*. Mitochondria are the parts of our cells responsible for producing the energy that cells need to carry out the necessary functions for survival. Within mitochondria, many chemical reactions occur to produce this energy in the form of adenosine triphosphate, or ATP. These chemical reactions require a number of nutrients and enzymes to proceed quickly and meet the body's needs. In people with fibromyalgia, the mitochondria don't function properly to produce the energy required by cells to function.[14-16] This is evident in studies showing decreased amounts of ATP in muscle and blood cells in people with fibromyalgia, both at rest and during exercise.[11,13,17] Research has shown that this mitochondrial dysfunction occurs because of a decreased number of mitochondria, as well as defects in the functioning of key mitochondrial enzymes. Deficiencies in nutrients required for the energy production process have also been identified.[11,14-16] When mitochondria aren't functioning properly, the body destroys them.[14] This destruction of malfunctioning parts is a normal bodily process; however, these mitochondria are eventually replaced with new mitochondria that also don't function well, and the cycle is repeated. A lack of proper energy production contributes to fatigue, pain, and cognitive symptoms. The good news is that with supplementation of nutrients that are suspected to be deficient, mitochondrial function and symptoms appear to improve.[15] We will discuss nutrients that support mitochondrial function in more detail in Chapter 11.

Some measures of inflammation in patients with fibromyalgia show higher than normal levels of inflammatory molecules within the blood and dysfunction in different parts of the immune system.[8,18-21] Studies show that some parts of the immune system are suppressed compared to people without fibromyalgia.[20-21] It is suspected that mitochondrial dysfunction, nutrient deficiencies, and an abnormal stress response all contribute to unhealthy levels of inflammation and an immune system that does not function as expected.[15,19]

As our understanding of how the body responds to stress develops, more research has been focused on the stress response in painful conditions such as fibromyalgia. The interplay between the nervous system and the body's response in the release of neurotransmitters and hormones can be complex, and we still have much to learn. Research performed specifically on people with fibromyalgia has shown that at rest, their bodies are in a high-stress state.[22,23] To the surprise of many researchers, the stress response in someone with fibromyalgia is less robust when exposed to a stressor than in someone without fibromyalgia.[22,23] This may be due to an overload of the stress response, meaning that the body of someone with fibromyalgia cannot mount an appropriate physical response to additional stress.[22] Researchers suspect that this high-stress state at rest and low response to stressors may be due to genetic differences in enzymes involved in the stress response, a history of high-stress events (trauma, abuse, etc.), and decreased sensitivity to messages stimulating an appropriate stress response.[24] Clinically, this dysfunction in the stress response can result in many of the symptoms associated with fibromyalgia, including fatigue, morning stiffness, sleep abnormalities, anxiety, Raynaud's phenomenon, and digestive symptoms.[22] We will discuss the stress response in more detail in Chapter 13.

Poor sleep is a very common problem for people with fibromyalgia. Sleep studies performed on people with fibromyalgia have shown deviations in what we would expect from a normal sleep cycle. In studies measuring brain waves during sleep, there is evidence of alpha brain waves intruding upon delta brain waves.[25] Alpha brain waves are the type present when you are awake or during periods of relaxation, such as meditation. Delta brain waves are present in deeper sleep, also called slow-wave sleep. In research comparing sleep in people with fibromyalgia to people with insomnia, there were significant differences in sleep measures between the two groups.[26] Both the fibromyalgia group and the insomnia group showed decreased total sleep time, decreased slow-wave (deeper) sleep, increased time to consistent sleep, and increased time spent awake through the night compared to people with no difficulty sleeping.[26] When comparing sleep between the fibromyalgia group and the insomnia group, researchers noticed that people with fibromyalgia had more slow-wave (deeper) sleep and shorter time to consistent sleep, but were awake for a similar amount of time during nighttime awakenings.[26] Specifically, people with fibromyalgia tended to wake more often through the night but were awake for shorter periods of time.[26] The abnormalities in brain wave activity during sleep and frequent nighttime awakenings make for poor sleep quality, which has been shown to increase pain levels and impair cognitive function in people with fibromyalgia.[27] Although pain levels can definitely affect sleep, research has shown that improving sleep quality decreases pain severity and improves cognitive function in people with fibromyalgia.[27,28] This is why sleep is the first aspect of your health we aim to improve with supplementation, after addressing the foundations of healing. See Chapter 9 for more details.

Fibromyalgia is often referred to as a disorder of centralized pain processing (also called central sensitization). Initially, researchers thought that the brain was more sensitive to pain signals travelling from the limbs of the body to the brain. It was suspected that these signals were amplified within the brain, resulting in higher pain intensity. Research investigating this theory compared brain imaging studies of people with fibromyalgia to people who did not have a painful condition.[29] In this research, there was evidence that the brain of a person with fibromyalgia reacts to lower stimulus levels in the form of a pressure sensation. Moreover, the brain interprets this signal as more painful, compared to people without a painful condition.[29] More recent research has shown that there may also be a dysfunction in communication between the areas of the brain that shut off pain signals.[30] This combination of amplified pain signals within the brain and an inability to turn such signals off may be at least partially due to the presence of inflammation within the brain and central nervous system. In studies measuring components in the fluid surrounding the brain and spinal cord, high levels of some inflammatory markers and low levels of some neurotransmitters (particularly serotonin and norepinephrine) were detected in people with fibromyalgia.[8,31] Inflammation and disrupted neurotransmitter balance within the brain and spinal cord help to explain the widespread nature of fibromyalgia symptoms and the dysfunction in pain signal processing observed.

Increasing attention is being dedicated to the role of digestion and gut bacteria in fibromyalgia. Research performed on gut bacteria composition in people with fibromyalgia has uncovered a strong correlation between small intestinal bacterial overgrowth (SIBO) and fibromyalgia.[32] It is possible that imbalances in different bacterial populations within the gut could be a causative factor for the symptoms and metabolic abnormalities noted in fibromyalgia. Various metabolites produced by common gut bacteria species have been linked to low levels of cortisol, vitamin D, tryptophan, serotonin, thyroid hormone, and melatonin; imbalances in all of which have been correlated with fibromyalgia.[32] Furthering the connection between gut bacteria imbalances and fibromyalgia, patients who achieved eradication of SIBO showed significant improvement in fibromyalgia symptoms.[32] Other research on this topic has uncovered distinct patterns in gut bacterial growth that seem to correlate with the symptoms and severity of fibromyalgia.[33] Stress has been identified as a potent disruptor of gut bacteria balance, and this may be the underlying factor that leads to imbalances.[31] Research in this area is ongoing and could provide new and exciting breakthroughs in fibromyalgia diagnosis and treatment.

As mentioned previously, there are a number of nutrient deficiencies that commonly occur in people with fibromyalgia. It is suspected that several of these deficiencies link to dysfunctions in the production of neurotransmitters within the brain or affect other physiologic processes that may contribute to the pain, fatigue, and cognitive symptoms associated with fibromyalgia.[34] At this time it is not clear whether there is an error in the absorption of these nutrients, their metabolism, or in both of these processes. Nutrient deficiencies that have been correlated with fibromyalgia include vitamin D, a number of amino acids, and coenzyme Q10.[34-36]

Hearing about all that is going wrong in your body can be discouraging. It can make you wonder how you will ever get better. From a medical standpoint, this information has been missing for years and is just what we need. When we understand what is going wrong in the body and begin to explore how it occurred, we can better tailor our treatments to address these dysfunctions to get the body functioning properly and heal the damage that has resulted.

## WHAT DOES SOMEONE WITH FIBROMYALGIA ACTUALLY EXPERIENCE?

Fibromyalgia is characterized by widespread body pain. This means that pain occurs above and below the waist, on both the right and left sides of the body.[37] Pain can be in the muscles, joints, or both. People with fibromyalgia describe the pain sensation differently. Some describe it as a dull ache, a burning sensation, a feeling of tension, or feeling sore all over, as though they had worked out the day before, even if they haven't. Along with the widespread pain, people with fibromyalgia also experience extreme fatigue.[38] This fatigue can be so severe that it is difficult to get out of bed or perform everyday activities, such as brushing your teeth or engaging in light household cleaning. Due to the sleep dysfunction that occurs with fibromyalgia, most people with the condition don't sleep well and don't wake up feeling refreshed.[38] The third core symptom of fibromyalgia is cognitive difficulty.[38] This includes difficulty remembering things, thinking clearly, paying attention for long periods of time, and engaging in conversation. *Fibro fog* is a term often used to describe the cognitive symptoms of fibromyalgia.

Along with the core symptoms of fibromyalgia, a variety of other symptoms commonly occur. These include:[38]

- Muscle weakness
- Digestive symptoms, such as abnormal stools, abdominal pain and cramps, constipation, diarrhea, nausea, heartburn, vomiting, loss of appetite
- Headaches or migraines
- Numbness, tingling, or itching
- Dizziness
- Insomnia
- Depression and anxiety or nervousness
- Chest pain
- Blurred vision, dry eyes
- Fever
- Oral symptoms including dry mouth, sores in the mouth, or loss/change of taste
- Wheezing or shortness of breath
- Raynaud's phenomenon
- Hives/welts, rash, sun sensitivity
- Ringing in the ears, hearing difficulty
- Seizures
- Easy bruising
- Hair loss
- Frequent urination, painful urination, bladder spasms

The huge variety of symptoms from all over the body is in part why fibromyalgia is difficult to diagnose and treat. It can be difficult for medical professionals to gather all of this information from patients in short visits. Fibromyalgia can also resemble many other conditions, making diagnosis tricky. See Chapter 3 for more information on conditions that can look like fibromyalgia.

## WHAT IS THE ROOT CAUSE OF FIBROMYALGIA?

I don't think we have the root cause of fibromyalgia completely figured out yet, but I do believe we have some key clues that can point us in a useful direction. We've discussed the underlying structural and functional abnormalities in fibromyalgia, and we've seen how they show up as an astonishing number of possible symptoms, but what is the one common thread that ties all of that together? What is the one thing we can target that can improve all of the abnormalities and symptoms related to fibromyalgia? My answer to these questions is the stress response.

In my work with fibromyalgia, I've seen it time and time again. The body tries to withstand the major stressors that are often experienced by someone with fibromyalgia, while maintaining an appropriate stress response. The problem is that on top of whatever major stressor you may have experienced (whether it's emotional trauma, a physical injury or accident, job loss, divorce, or death of a loved one), everyday life still happens, and you are still exposed to many smaller stressors all the time. Your body doesn't have time to fully recover and recuperate from these stressors. This lack of time for healing combined with a genetic predisposition is the perfect storm. Over time, stress harms the basic functioning of the body and causes damage to tissues responsible for maintaining the stress response.

The body responds to all stressors with the same basic stress response. The stress can be physical, mental, or emotional, but physiologically it's all the same to your body. No matter the type of stress, it triggers the same cascade of reactions. Stress wreaks havoc on the body. It triggers the body to use more resources over a shorter period of time. This can be seen as nutrient deficiencies and abnormalities in energy production, with resources being depleted faster than they can be replaced. Stress causes immune system suppression and generates inflammation all over the body, affecting the brain, mitochondria, and muscles. Stress occupies your mind constantly, despite your best efforts to relax and rest. It causes your muscles to be ready to respond to danger at a moment's notice, with a constant state of contraction and low activity, rather than rest. Many of the dysfunctions identified in fibromyalgia can be linked directly to the stress response. Fibromyalgia appears to be a full-body presentation of *burnout*, where the body can no longer sustain an active stress response.

So how do we heal your body from the symptoms that plague you? In the treatment section of this book, we will work to create the basic healing environment your body needs, while also training your body to respond to stress differently. This is achieved by continually showing your body that it is safe and has everything it needs to survive. You will practice training your body to respond appropriately when stress does occur and to turn off the stress response once the stress is gone. We will repair the damage done by the chronic stress response, and we will heal the mind and the body.

## KEY POINTS

- Your symptoms are not made up or all in your head.
- Fibromyalgia has a physiologic basis, with a number of physical abnormalities identified.
- Core symptoms of fibromyalgia include pain, fatigue, and cognitive dysfunction (fibro fog).
- There are a number of other symptoms that can occur with fibromyalgia.
- The root cause of fibromyalgia is not yet known, but likely involves abnormalities in the way the body responds to stress.

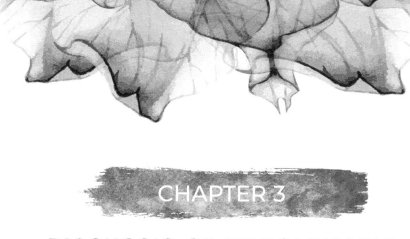

# CHAPTER 3

# DIAGNOSIS OF FIBROMYALGIA

Now that you know what fibromyalgia is, the next question is, how is it diagnosed? The proper diagnosis of fibromyalgia is a controversial topic in medicine. Part of this controversy stems from the fact that our conventional medical system is broken up into specialties, with little attention given to whole body medicine. Fibromyalgia can fall under the supervision of multiple specialties, with no one individual allotting enough time to consider all aspects of your body and your symptoms. This is in no way the fault of medical professionals but is simply the way our medical system has developed over time. The other difficulty with fibromyalgia is that there are no *objective* methods to determine whether a patient has the condition. This means that beyond your reports of symptoms, health care providers have no reliable blood tests or imaging to confirm the diagnosis. Further complicating this matter is the fact that symptoms of fibromyalgia can overlap with those of a number of other conditions.

For the reasons listed above, a diagnosis of fibromyalgia is only made once symptoms have been present for at least three months.[38] Previously, it was recommended that all other possible causes of symptoms be ruled out before diagnosing fibromyalgia; however, this recommendation no longer stands.[39] In 2016, the diagnostic criteria for fibromyalgia were revised to state that as long as the fibromyalgia criteria were met, a diagnosis of fibromyalgia could be made regardless of other conditions present.[39] As you will read in Chapter 5, there are a number of other conditions that tend to occur more often in people with fibromyalgia. If at any time in the diagnostic process it is discovered that you have another condition that may be contributing to the symptoms you are experiencing, you can still be diagnosed with fibromyalgia, but treatment of the co-occurring condition should also be initiated.

## OLD METHOD OF DIAGNOSING FIBROMYALGIA: TENDER POINT EXAMINATION

In 1990, a group of researchers developed the American College of Rheumatology 1990 fibromyalgia diagnostic criteria, which included the tender point examination.[37] This examination involves applying pressure to 18 specific points on the torso, both sides of the body, and above and below the waist. To meet the criteria for fibromyalgia, a person must experience widespread pain, classified as tenderness at 11 or more of the 18 points.[37] Widespread pain is defined as pain on the left and right side of the body, pain above and below the waist, and pain in the neck or mid-back area of the spine, in the front of the chest, or in the low back.[37]

While a physical exam can be a great way to gather information about a condition, a few issues arose with the tender point examination. To perform the tender point examination according to the standard, 4kg of pressure must be applied using the thumb or the first two or three fingers.[37] The appropriate pressure to apply is difficult to determine and subject to variability between practitioners and between different measurement times by the same practitioner. It was determined that many practitioners were not using the tender point examination in practice, partly because many had not been trained in how to perform it.[38] In addition, the performance of this exam can be incredibly uncomfortable for patients. In research performed on this form of diagnosis for fibromyalgia, the tender point exam tended to misdiagnose fibromyalgia in men.[3]

The most important criticism of the tender point examination is that it does not take into account other fibromyalgia symptoms.[38] There is no evaluation of sleep dysfunction, brain fog, fatigue, or other bodily symptoms beyond pain. In light of these downfalls, while the examination may still be useful, it should not be the sole method for diagnosing fibromyalgia.

## NEW METHOD OF DIAGNOSING FIBROMYALGIA: WPI-SSS

In 2010, a different group of researchers developed the American College of Rheumatology 2010 preliminary fibromyalgia diagnostic criteria, which involves the widespread pain index and symptom severity score (WPI-SSS).[38] The WPI-SSS is a questionnaire that can be filled out in-office by an individual with suspected fibromyalgia. Additionally, the WPI-SSS can be used to monitor symptoms after the initial diagnosis has been made.[38]

On the widespread pain index portion of the WPI-SSS, patients are asked to check off all the areas in which they have experienced pain over the past week. This portion of the questionnaire is similar to the tender point examination for locations of pain.[38] The WPI portion is scored from 0 to 19, with one point allocated for each painful area checked off.[38]

The symptom severity score portion of the WPI-SSS is broken up into two parts. In part 2a, patients are asked to rate the severity of three core symptoms of fibromyalgia over the past week.[38] The ratings for fatigue, waking unrefreshed, and cognitive symptoms occur on a 0 to 3 point scale, with 0 assigned to no problem with the symptom and 3 assigned to severe difficulty with the symptom. For part 2a, the score is calculated by adding up the points allocated to the severity of each symptom (not the number of check marks in the section).[38]

Part 2b of the symptom severity score inventories the other symptoms that commonly occur with fibromyalgia.[38] In this section, patients check off the symptoms they have experienced within the past week. There are 41 symptoms listed here. The scoring of this section is a bit tricky. If none of the listed symptoms have been experienced, the score is 0. If 1–10 symptoms have been experienced, the score is 1. For 11–24 symptoms, the score is 2. Finally, if 25 or more symptoms have been checked off in part 2b, the score is 3.[38]

To finish scoring this questionnaire, the scores from parts 2a and 2b are added. The score for the SSS section can range from 0–12.[38] The WPI score stays as previously calculated. There are two ways to meet the new diagnostic criteria for fibromyalgia. In the first scoring scenario, the pain score is high, with a WPI score of at least 7 and an SS score of at least 5.[38] In the second scenario, the pain score is lower, but the symptom severity score is high, with a WPI equal to 3–6 and an SS score of at least 9.[38] In both scoring scenarios, the symptoms must have been present for at least three months, without other conditions that could explain the pain (unless already appropriately treated).

I recommend doing the WPI-SSS with your health care provider, as the scoring can be challenging, and it is helpful to be able to ask questions as you go through it. As you can see, the WPI-SSS is very thorough and takes into account many more symptoms of fibromyalgia than just pain. I also find this tool useful to measure progress over time, along with the fibromyalgia impact questionnaire, to get a consistent measure of how your symptoms are affecting your everyday activities. Drawbacks of the WPI-SSS include the lack of objective measurements (lab results or imaging) to help confirm a fibromyalgia diagnosis and the emotional reaction that can occur when you see your scores. Seeing your symptoms laid out on paper can be scary and discouraging, especially before you have received any treatment. It's normal and perfectly valid to feel this way. With treatment and dedication on your part, seeing your scores come down will be rewarding and will encourage you to continue on your health journey.

## OTHER CONDITIONS THAT LOOK LIKE FIBROMYALGIA

There are a number of conditions with symptoms similar to the core symptoms of fibromyalgia. It's important to also consider these conditions when making a fibromyalgia diagnosis, since there are no blood tests or imaging studies that can definitively determine whether you have fibromyalgia. Many of these other conditions have fatigue, pain, cognitive dysfunction, or a combination of symptoms that also occur with fibromyalgia. A diagnosis of one of these other conditions would change the treatment approach in most cases. As mentioned previously, a diagnosis of fibromyalgia can be made if you meet the criteria for fibromyalgia, but other conditions that could be contributing to your symptoms should be appropriately investigated and treated. For a thorough list of conditions that can look like fibromyalgia, consult the Additional Resources section or download your own copy here: https:// resources.flourishingwithfibromyalgia.com/fibromyalgia-resource-guide, and speak with your health care provider about a proper diagnostic workup for your symptoms.

## POSSIBLE FUTURE DIAGNOSTIC TECHNIQUES

As mentioned previously, it is ideal to have some objective measurement of a condition in the form of a blood test or imaging. The lack of such a measurement is one of the difficulties in diagnosing fibromyalgia. The good news is that there are a number of exciting possibilities in the future of fibromyalgia diagnosis. Research in this area is ongoing.

Possibilities for future diagnostic techniques in assisting with fibromyalgia diagnosis could include measurements of any of the abnormalities discussed in Chapter 2. The most likely options include genetic testing, blood testing, brain imaging, measures of mitochondrial function, and tests mapping the gut microflora. For a specific diagnostic procedure to be widely adopted in medicine, the technique should give one result when a person has fibromyalgia (we call this a *positive* result) and a different result when a person does not have fibromyalgia (we call this a *negative* result). This is not always possible, but it is ideal. We also want a test to be relatively inexpensive and easy to perform.

Although we can identify a number of different abnormalities in the body of someone with fibromyalgia, the difficulty lies in distinguishing fibromyalgia from other similar conditions. Many of the abnormalities discussed in Chapter 2 have also been linked to other conditions. That is to say, they are not unique to fibromyalgia. With further research, it is likely that we will uncover a specific pattern of measurable abnormalities in fibromyalgia, and this will help immensely with diagnosis. Our understanding of fibromyalgia has come a long way, and I am confident that we will find an objective measurement unique to this condition.

## KEY POINTS

- Tender point examination is the old method for diagnosing fibromyalgia.
- Widespread pain index and symptom severity score (WPI-SSS) is the new method for diagnosing fibromyalgia.
- Both the tender point examination and WPI-SSS have pros and cons.
- It is important to investigate any other conditions that can look like fibromyalgia, as these conditions are often treated differently than fibromyalgia.
- There are many possibilities for objective testing options in the future of fibromyalgia diagnosis.

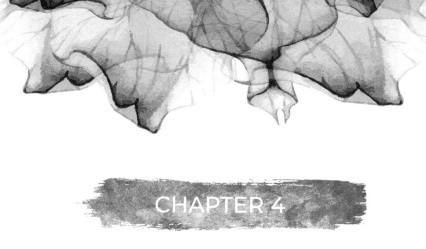

# CHAPTER 4

# LABS TO CONSIDER

We've discussed what fibromyalgia is and how to properly diagnose it, which if you recall does not include any specific lab testing to confirm a fibromyalgia diagnosis. So why is there a whole chapter on lab testing? There are a number of lab tests that are useful in determining whether the symptoms you are experiencing are due to fibromyalgia or a condition that looks like fibromyalgia. Lab testing is also useful when we are sure of a fibromyalgia diagnosis, as these labs can give us more information on what is going wrong in the body and contributing to your symptoms. This information allows for more targeted treatments.

I have organized the lab tests into categories based on what type of sample is tested (e.g., blood, breath, stool). In each category, I will describe when I find this test most useful in my practice. Some health care practitioners do not have access to or are not familiar with all of these testing options. For example, naturopathic doctors in Ontario cannot order imaging, and some medical doctors may not be familiar with the functional medicine testing I will discuss. In some cases, a health care provider can determine where you could access a test and refer you, if necessary. In some parts of the world, certain tests may not be available, but there may be alternatives.

Your health care provider will be able to determine which tests are most relevant based on the symptoms you are experiencing. For example, some conditions have characteristic symptoms, and if you are not experiencing these symptoms then it is very unlikely you have that condition, and it would be a waste of time and money to send you for testing related to the condition in question. If you find that reading this chapter feels like reading a foreign language, do not stress about it. You will not lose out on the information later on if you skim this chapter or skip it altogether. This chapter is intended to provide you with information on what should be investigated in relation to your symptoms, because you deserve to know what is happening in your care. Your health care provider will be able to guide you through this process and should answer any questions you have.

## BASIC BLOOD TESTING

Blood testing is the most basic testing we will discuss and in general, the easiest to access. We use these blood tests most often to rule out conditions that may look like fibromyalgia, as discussed in Chapter 3. If what you are experiencing is truly fibromyalgia, the basic blood tests will come back normal. Do not let this discourage you. If you are experiencing symptoms, there is a physical reason for it. Your experience is valid and deserves recognition. The challenge is whether we can find this abnormality on a lab test. This is a limitation of our ability to measure different processes in the body, not a reflection of your experience or the validity of your symptoms.

## Nutrient Deficiencies

Evaluation for nutrient deficiencies is often included in initial routine blood work to investigate fatigue and pain. One of the most useful tests in this category is a complete blood count (CBC), which inventories the numbers, sizes, and types of red and white blood cells, as well as platelets, present in your blood. The CBC can give clues about anemias, cancers, infections, and nutrient deficiencies. Pairing the CBC with a measure of RBC (red blood cell) folate level, vitamin B12, and tests for iron status gives us further information regarding nutritional status. Tests for iron status can include serum iron, transferrin saturation, ferritin (measure of iron stores), and serum total iron-binding capacity (TIBC). In addition, testing 25-hydroxyvitamin D helps to determine if vitamin D deficiency is contributing to symptoms. Since vitamin D deficiency is so common in Canada, most provincial health plans do not cover the cost of the test, resulting in an out-of-pocket expense for patients. Another possible contributor to pain is magnesium deficiency. Unfortunately, there is no reliable lab test to determine whether magnesium is deficient. If a magnesium deficiency is suspected, the best way to determine whether this is contributing to symptoms is to supplement with magnesium for a period of time and monitor for symptom improvement.

## Organ Function

Tests evaluating the function of both the liver and the kidneys are simple to obtain and can help provide evidence for a specific diagnosis. For example, if hepatitis is suspected to be contributing to symptoms, basic liver function tests can be performed. Liver function tests can include liver enzyme levels in the blood, such as alanine aminotransferase (ALT), aspartate transaminase (AST), alkaline phosphatase (ALP), and bilirubin. When the liver is damaged, these liver enzymes leak out of the liver cells and into your blood. Bilirubin is formed when red blood cells are broken down, and it is your liver's job to get rid of the waste products. Your health care provider may also choose to measure hepatitis virus antibodies, albumin, and international normalized ratio (INR). Albumin is a protein present in the blood that is produced by the liver and can indicate whether the liver is functioning properly. INR is a measure of the blood's clotting ability. Clotting factors are proteins in the blood that play a role in blood clotting. Some clotting factors are produced in the liver and can provide clues as to how the liver is functioning.

Kidney function testing often includes a measurement of creatinine and estimated glomerular filtration rate (eGFR) in the blood. It may also include a urinalysis, since it is the kidney's job to produce urine. Kidney function can be diminished as a result of a number of conditions, including systemic lupus erythematosus (SLE) and advanced diabetes mellitus, among others.

## Inflammatory Markers

The typical inflammatory markers measured in the investigation of fibromyalgia include erythrocyte sedimentation rate (ESR) and C-reactive protein (CRP). Both of these measures tend to be normal in fibromyalgia but can be elevated in conditions that mimic fibromyalgia. An elevation in either ESR or CRP should prompt further investigation for rheumatoid arthritis, polymyalgia rheumatica, and other inflammatory conditions.

## Infections

We've already discussed a CBC and hepatitis viral antibodies as possible tests to provide clues as to whether an infection is contributing to symptoms. Other possible infectious causes of symptoms include human immunodeficiency virus (HIV), Epstein–Barr virus (EBV), Lyme disease, tuberculosis, and mould and mycotoxin illness.

Testing for Lyme disease is more complicated than the basic blood tests and will be discussed in the *Advanced Blood Testing* section of this chapter. Testing for tuberculosis cannot be done via blood testing and will be discussed in the *Other Testing* section of this chapter. Unfortunately, mould and mycotoxin illnesses have no reliable testing method available for diagnosis at this time. This diagnosis is made based on clinical symptoms and a history of exposure or suspected exposure to mould. Basic blood tests that can be performed for infectious causes include antibodies and viral load testing for HIV and testing for EBV infection. The initial test for EBV usually involves what is called a monospot test. The monospot test requires a small sample of blood taken from your fingertip. If further testing is required, a blood sample may be taken from your vein to test for EBV antibodies.

## Endocrine Disorders

Basic blood testing can also be used to determine whether diabetes mellitus or thyroid conditions are contributing to your symptoms. Some of these tests can also point us in the direction of Cushing syndrome; however, further testing and referral to a specialist may be required to make this diagnosis definitively.

To investigate blood sugar regulation, fasting blood glucose (FBG), hemoglobin A1c (HbA1c), and insulin provide the most information. Fasting blood glucose gives us a blood sugar measurement at the time of the blood draw, whereas HbA1c gives us an idea of blood sugar levels over the past three months. Some health care providers do not include a measurement of insulin; however, I find it useful for detecting insulin resistance prior to the body reaching a level of dysfunction classified as type 2 diabetes mellitus. Investigation for diabetes may also include a urinalysis, which is discussed further in the *Urine Tests* section of this chapter.

Basic testing for both hypothyroidism and hyperthyroidism includes testing thyroid-stimulating hormone (TSH), free T3, and free T4. TSH is the hormone that comes from the brain to signal to the thyroid that it needs to produce thyroid hormones. Free T3 and free T4 are measures of the thyroid hormones that act on cells in the body. In Canada, most medical doctors will only order TSH as an initial screen for thyroid dysfunction. In my practice, I test for all three thyroid-related hormones, as it is possible for TSH to come up normal while free T3 and free T4 show dysfunction in the thyroid gland. As discussed in the *Autoimmune Disorders* section of this chapter, some thyroid conditions are autoimmune in nature, and there are antibodies that may be included in evaluating thyroid function through blood testing. See the *Autoimmune Disorders* section for more information.

Cortisol is another basic blood test that can be performed. Cortisol may be measured to investigate Cushing syndrome or Addison's disease. Addison's disease is both an autoimmune and an endocrine condition. With an abnormal cortisol level in the blood, further testing and referral to a specialist may be required.

## Autoimmune Disorders

Autoimmune disorders can be difficult to diagnose and may require referral to a specialist, depending on what type of health care practitioner you are working with. Some antibody tests can point us more clearly towards one autoimmune disease, compared to others. Conditions that typically require referral to a specialist include systemic lupus erythematosus (SLE), Addison's disease (discussed in the *Endocrine Conditions* section of this chapter), and myasthenia gravis.

As discussed in the *Endocrine Conditions* section of this chapter, thyroid conditions can be caused by an autoimmune process in the body. Adding thyroid peroxidase antibodies (TPO), thyroglobulin antibodies (TGAb), thyroid-stimulating immunoglobulin (TSI), and thyroid-binding inhibitory immunoglobulin (TBII) to a lab requisition may be helpful in determining whether the thyroid dysfunction is caused by autoimmunity. These tests are not always performed because the results may not change the treatment options. Naturally, autoimmune thyroid conditions are often treated differently that non-autoimmune thyroid conditions.

The inflammatory markers ESR and CRP discussed previously may be elevated in cases of rheumatoid arthritis. Additional testing could include rheumatoid factor and anti-cyclic citrullinated peptide (anti-CCP) antibodies. As discussed in the *Imaging* section of this chapter, X-rays may also be ordered to determine the extent of joint damage in rheumatoid arthritis.

Systemic lupus erythematosus (SLE, also known as lupus) and myasthenia gravis are conditions that can be challenging to diagnose and often require investigation by a specialist. A number of antibodies can be associated with SLE, including antinuclear antibodies (ANA), anti-dsDNA, and cardiolipin antibodies. Additional testing that can provide more information regarding suspected SLE includes CBC, kidney function, liver function, and urinalysis, as discussed elsewhere in this chapter. Myasthenia gravis may show elevated acetylcholine receptor antibodies on lab work; however, this is not a test that is ordered by most health care practitioners.

## Muscle Testing

Some conditions have muscle pain as a symptom because the body is breaking down muscle tissue, or there has been an injury to muscle tissue. These conditions can present with widespread muscle pain. All of the following tests are expected to be normal in fibromyalgia but could be abnormal in a number of other conditions. Testing for muscle breakdown can include creatine kinase, aldolase, ALT, and AST. You may remember ALT and AST from the *Organ Function* section of this chapter, as these enzymes are present in both muscle cells and liver cells.

## ADVANCED BLOOD TESTING

Testing that falls into this category is either functional medicine testing or blood testing that is not typically ordered by general health care practitioners. Some of the tests discussed in the Basic Blood Testing category could also fall into the advanced testing category (tests that may require referral to a specialist); however, these were included in the discussion of basic testing for completeness and relevance to the topic at hand.

## Food Sensitivity Testing

Food sensitivities are different from food allergies and food intolerances. Food allergies are reactions that occur within minutes of eating a particular food and can be very serious. Examples of food allergies include allergies to peanuts or seafood. Symptoms related to a food allergy often require emergency medical care and may include hives, skin rashes, difficulty breathing, swelling of the tongue or lips, stomach pain, nausea, or diarrhea, among others.[40-41] Food allergies are caused by a part of your immune system called IgE antibodies that react with a specific food. Food sensitivities differ from food allergies in that they involve a different part of the immune system, called IgG antibodies. Symptoms related to food sensitivities are delayed and can take hours or days to show up. Because of the delay between when a food is consumed and when symptoms of food sensitivities occur, pinpointing the causes can be difficult. In contrast, food intolerances do not involve the immune system at all. Instead, they are caused by the deficiency or complete absence of a specific enzyme required to digest and absorb a particular food component. An example of food intolerance is lactose intolerance, which occurs when there is a deficiency in lactase, the enzyme required to break apart lactose.

Food sensitivities can cause a number of symptoms throughout the body, including fever, fatigue, sweating, feeling weak, skin itching and rashes, mood and memory disturbances, migraines, asthma symptoms, joint pain, or muscle stiffness. Digestive symptoms are also common with food sensitivities and may include abdominal pain, gas, bloating, nausea, vomiting, or diarrhea.[42] Many of these symptoms overlap with fibromyalgia and can make the symptoms of fibromyalgia much worse.

There are two ways to investigate food sensitivities. You can either do an elimination diet (discussed in detail in Chapter 7) or complete a test for food sensitivities. The food sensitivity test I use in my practice requires a small sample of blood collected at a lab. This blood sample is used to measure the levels of IgG antibodies in response to a number of different foods. There are several different panels, depending on which foods you would like tested. Different tests will likely present the results differently. The results of the test I use are presented in three categories. Foods that produce lower levels of IgG antibodies are considered *non-reactive* foods. Foods that produce a moderate level of IgG antibodies are considered *borderline*. The last category is foods that produce elevated IgG antibody levels. These foods are considered *reactive* foods. I generally advise my patients to avoid the foods that fall into the borderline and reactive categories, as these are generating inflammation within the body. Avoidance of all borderline and reactive foods is not always possible if these categories contain a large number of foods. Always seek individualized dietary advice based on your food sensitivity results to ensure you are not excluding important nutrients from your diet.

## Lyme Disease Testing

There is a lot of controversy in the area of Lyme disease testing, and there is much room for improvement in cost-effective testing techniques. Conventionally, most medical doctors will order a blood test to screen for antibodies to *Borrelia burgdorferi*, the bacteria that causes Lyme disease. This test is called the enzyme-linked immunosorbent assay, or ELISA. ELISA should be combined with a Western blot test to minimize the chances of a falsely negative result; however, the Western blot test is usually ordered to confirm a positive result obtained on the ELISA test. The ELISA test can be falsely negative in the early stage of Lyme disease, when the body has not produced enough antibodies to obtain a positive result. This means that your test result comes back negative, but you do in fact have Lyme disease. False negatives with the ELISA test are estimated to occur in about 50% of tests run, and it is estimated that the Western blot test is only about 80% accurate in detecting Lyme disease.[43] In addition, there are a number of co-infections that commonly occur with a *Borrelia burgdorferi* infection that are not tested for using conventional Lyme disease testing methods.

Since the accuracy of the standard conventional testing for Lyme disease is abysmal at best and co-infections are not investigated, it may be worthwhile to consider alternative testing for Lyme disease. There are a number of private labs conducting Lyme disease testing. I typically opt for the Armin Labs TickPlex test, but this is not the only option available. The TickPlex test measures IgG and IgM antibodies to *Borrelia burgdorferi* and a number of common co-infecting bacteria in a blood sample.[44] The downside to this test is that it is expensive.

## Sex Hormone Testing

In some cases, symptoms point towards a sex hormone imbalance that may be contributing to pain, fatigue, cognitive symptoms, difficulty sleeping, painful menses, and mood changes. Investigating and correcting these imbalances can make treatments selected to address fibromyalgia symptoms much more effective or even prevent the need for further fibromyalgia treatment. Sex hormones include follicle-stimulating hormone (FSH), luteinizing hormone (LH), estrogen, and progesterone, as well as free and total testosterone.

Testing of sex hormones can occur in a number of different ways, including blood testing, salivary testing, and urine testing. I use blood and urine testing in my practice. This section includes information on blood testing for sex hormones. See the *Urine Tests* section for a description of urinary hormone testing.

Blood testing of sex hormones falls into the advanced testing category because in a menstruating female (a female who gets her period), testing on specific days of the cycle gives us more useful results. This means that it may be necessary to track your menstrual cycle and have several lab requisitions to get all of the hormone testing completed. To accurately track your cycle, count the first day of your menstrual period as day 1 of your cycle. Your cycle ends the day before your next period (the first day of bleeding of your next period is day 1 of your next cycle). When performing blood testing of sex hormones in my practice, I recommend my patients get their estradiol (a type of estrogen), LH, and FSH levels tested on day 3 of their cycle. I provide my patients with another requisition for progesterone, free testosterone, and total testosterone testing, which should be measured seven days before your next period. This method of testing is trickier with irregular periods, but it can be done. Absent periods may require additional testing beyond what is discussed in this section and are beyond the scope of this book. Please discuss this with your health care provider.

## IMAGING STUDIES

Imaging may be required to investigate for specific diagnoses or assess the extent of a disease. Examples of imaging studies that may be performed in the investigation of fibromyalgia include ultrasound, X-ray, magnetic resonance imaging (MRI), and computerized tomography (CT) scans. Imaging may be performed to investigate for abdominal and digestive conditions, arthritis, lung conditions, and multiple sclerosis, among many others. Imaging does not provide any information about fibromyalgia specifically but can help determine if there are any other conditions occurring in addition to fibromyalgia.

## OTHER TESTS

There are a number of other tests that may be relevant to the investigation of fibromyalgia, such as nerve testing. Nerve testing would be used if pain seems to be related to nerves, or you are experiencing abnormal sensations such as numbness or tingling. Testing of sputum (the mucus spit up when coughing) may be completed if tuberculosis or a respiratory infection is suspected. Finally, a sleep study (termed polysomnography) may be performed to rule out sleep apnea. Patients with fibromyalgia experience dysfunction in their sleep cycles and often show abnormalities on a sleep study.[25–26]

## URINE TESTS

### Urinalysis

As discussed in the *Basic Blood Tests* section, a urinalysis may be added to the basic blood tests to help determine whether any other conditions are present. A urinalysis is easy to complete and can provide information regarding kidney function, infection, and blood sugar regulation. Urine testing can be performed to measure cortisol and investigate some of the more complex endocrine conditions; however, this is not reported on a basic urinalysis and must be requested specifically by your health care provider.

## Organic Acids Test

I find the organic acids test to be one of the most useful tests in fibromyalgia. I use this test once we are sure that we are dealing with fibromyalgia. As described in the name, this test measures organic acids in a urine sample. Organic acids are compounds excreted in the urine at higher concentrations than are present in the blood. These compounds can be measured to provide information about different metabolic processes in the body.

When a metabolic process is not functioning optimally, it may be due to an enzyme that isn't functioning as it should or lack of a nutrient required for the enzyme to do its job. When this occurs, there is a buildup of a component along the pathway that provides information about which enzyme is not functioning properly. The specific test I use in my practice includes markers that give information regarding the health of the intestinal populations of bacteria, fungi, and yeasts, mitochondrial function, neurotransmitter levels, vitamin and mineral levels (including B vitamins and coenzyme Q10, which are important in energy production), oxidative stress, and measures of detoxification efficiency.[45] From this report, I am able to target a treatment plan to the individual person in front of me much more effectively, as we have evidence of where exactly the body is not functioning well.

Note: This test is a functional medicine test, and your health care provider may not be familiar with it.

## Urinary Hormone Test

There are a number of labs that provide urinary analysis of hormones. Some labs combine urinary sex hormone testing with salivary cortisol testing to get a better idea of how the HPA (hypothalamic–pituitary–adrenal) axis is functioning.[46] Urinary hormone testing provides a more thorough examination of the sex hormones compared to blood hormone testing. This type of testing includes measurements of the three forms of estrogen, progesterone, testosterone, and DHEA, as well as the adrenal hormone cortisol and its metabolites.[47] Using the results of this test, we can see where in the hormonal pathways imbalances are occurring and how that is affecting hormones in other parts of the pathway, allowing for a targeted treatment plan to correct the imbalance.

When urinary hormone testing is combined with salivary cortisol testing, we can examine the cortisol awakening response (CAR). The cortisol awakening response is the normal rise of cortisol levels within 60 minutes of waking. Measurements taken at 30 and 60 minutes after waking can provide us with information about whether cortisol levels are rising normally or abnormally after waking.[47] When combined with urine testing, we can also assess how cortisol is being metabolized within the body.

Research performed on cortisol levels in people with fibromyalgia has had mixed results. Some studies have shown low levels of cortisol in people with fibromyalgia, whereas others have shown normal or high levels.[48-51] Other studies have taken cortisol measurements one step further and determined that people with fibromyalgia may have dysfunctional cortisol cycles throughout the day.[52-53] Normally, cortisol levels are highest in the morning and slowly drop during the day. Some research has shown that cortisol levels in people with fibromyalgia are low in the morning and higher later in the day.[52-53] Cortisol and melatonin are opposing hormones in a delicate cycle regulating sleep response and daytime functioning. If cortisol levels are high, melatonin levels are typically low. A dysfunctional cortisol–melatonin cycle may partially explain the sleep difficulty associated with fibromyalgia, especially if cortisol levels are higher later in the day. We will discuss the stress response and how it affects treatment in more detail in Chapter 13.

Note: This test is a functional medicine test, and your health care provider may not be familiar with it.

## BREATH TESTS

The utilization of breath tests relates to the digestive symptoms that commonly occur with fibromyalgia. There are two main types of breath tests I use with my fibromyalgia patients. The first test is performed fairly regularly in conventional medicine. It is the breath test for *Helicobacter pylori* (termed *H. pylori* for short). *H. pylori* is a bacteria that can live in your stomach and increases the risk of stomach ulcers.[54] While *H. pylori* is not specifically linked to fibromyalgia, it can cause a number of the digestive symptoms commonly experienced in fibromyalgia. Since stomach ulcers are highly unpleasant, it is worthwhile to exclude this as a contributor.

The second breath test I use with my patients is the small intestinal bacterial overgrowth (SIBO) breath test. Unlike *H. pylori*, SIBO is strongly linked to fibromyalgia and suspected to be a causative factor in some cases.[32] Medical doctors can order the SIBO breath test, but this does not occur frequently in my experience. For a more thorough description of SIBO, see Chapter 5.

## STOOL TESTS

The utility of stool testing is again related to the high prevalence of digestive symptoms in fibromyalgia patients. There are two main types of stool testing I use in my practice. The first is the basic stool ova and parasite test that can be ordered from most laboratories. Medical doctors do order this test, and at times it is very useful. Ova and parasites can be picked up while travelling or when contaminated food and/or water are consumed. This type of infection is less common in Canada and the United States but could occur from consuming untreated lake water, for example. The stool ova and parasite test is an easy and inexpensive first step in stool testing.

If further stool testing is warranted, I use a comprehensive stool analysis test. This test uses a stool sample to determine which populations of bacteria, parasites, yeasts, and fungi are present in the intestines.[55] The test I use goes one step further and determines what medications and natural antimicrobials the pathogens are sensitive to. This information prevents us from treating with an agent that won't kill what we intend it to. This test is also helpful in determining if healthy bacterial populations need to be supported to help balance out the gut microflora.

Note: This test is a functional medicine test, and your health care provider may not be familiar with it.

## KEY POINTS

- There are many testing options that can help provide more information about dysfunction within the body in fibromyalgia.
- These tests can help guide treatment, but answers aren't guaranteed.

- These tests can be expensive, so if it comes to covering your basic necessities or taking a test, always choose the basic necessities.
- Work with a health care provider to determine which tests will provide the most information based on your symptoms.

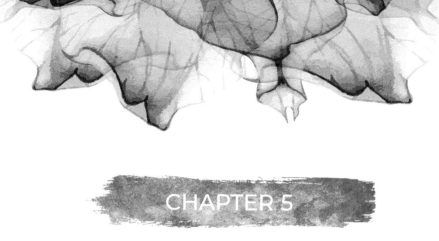

# CHAPTER 5

# CONDITIONS THAT COMMONLY OCCUR WITH FIBROMYALGIA

Many of the lab tests discussed in Chapter 4 will provide information on conditions that commonly occur alongside fibromyalgia. Part of the complexity of treating fibromyalgia is due to the number of other conditions that commonly occur with it. This can contribute to the wide variety of symptoms present all over the body. For health care providers, it can be difficult to determine which symptoms are caused by fibromyalgia and which are caused by another condition. It is difficult to address these conditions without the addition of more medications unless the root cause of fibromyalgia is addressed.

## NUTRIENT DEFICIENCIES

We discussed nutrient deficiencies in Chapter 3. However, nutrient deficiencies can also occur once a diagnosis of fibromyalgia has been given. The most common nutrient deficiencies that are associated with widespread pain are deficiencies in iron, vitamin B12, magnesium, and vitamin D.[8,11,35,56] Since deficiencies in these nutrients can cause symptoms that overlap with fibromyalgia, it is important that they are addressed. As discussed previously, deficiencies in several amino acids and coenzyme Q10 are also likely in fibromyalgia, but we have no way of testing for deficiencies in these nutrients.[14–16,34,36]

Nutrient deficiencies can occur for a number of reasons, including poor diet, depletion from medication, an increased need for the nutrient (due to stress, for example), poor absorption despite adequate dietary intake, or possibly a genetic defect in the pathways involving the nutrient. It is not always possible to identify the cause of a deficiency, especially in the case of genetic differences in nutrient pathways. However, it is possible to identify whether a medication is depleting a nutrient. I have included a resource called *Mytavin* in the *Additional Resources* section that your health care provider can use to determine if a medication is contributing to a deficiency.[57] If this is the case, it is ideal to discontinue the medication if possible. If the medication must be taken, then the appropriate nutrient should be supplemented for as long as the medication is taken. If a medication depletes a number of nutrients, a good-quality multivitamin may be a better option.

### Iron Deficiency

If a deficiency in iron is identified on blood work, it can take some time to increase iron storage levels. Remember, iron can be deficient even if you are not anemic. The storage form of iron in the body is called ferritin on lab reports. In some individuals, replenishing iron stores can take up to a year or more. It is important to consult with a health care provider prior to starting an iron supplement. Since iron is stored in the body, it is possible to reach toxic levels, and this can be dangerous to your health. In addition, some people do not tolerate iron supplements well and experience stomach irritation, diarrhea, constipation, nausea, or vomiting.[58]

There are two forms of iron in food: heme and non-heme. Heme iron comes from animal sources and is better absorbed by the human body.[58] Non-heme iron is the only form of iron present in plant sources and is not absorbed as well as heme iron. This means that you need to consume a higher amount of non-heme iron to raise iron stores, compared to the amount of heme iron you would need to consume.[58] In my practice, when adding an iron supplement I choose a supplement containing heme iron where possible. I find that we can dose the supplement lower, it is tolerated better by patients, and ferritin levels increase faster than with a non-heme iron supplement. Supplements containing heme iron can be harder to find, but they are available.

If an iron deficiency is identified, but your lab work does not show anemia, a daily dose of 50–75mg of elemental iron would be enough to bring ferritin levels to within normal in the general population.[59] If lab work does show an iron deficiency anemia, a dose of 150–200mg of daily elemental iron may be necessary to replenish iron stores within the body.[59] Iron supplements should always be taken with food to minimize digestive upset and increase absorption of the supplement. Since the lifespan of a red blood cell is 120 days, it takes at least three to four months for ferritin levels to change on a lab report. As a result, it is not worth retesting labs until supplementation has been consistent for three to six months.

Adverse effects of iron supplementation are fairly common and can be very uncomfortable. With fibromyalgia, your body also tends to be more sensitive to supplements in general. As with any new addition in fibromyalgia, you want to start at a low dose and slowly work your way up. Always listen to your body. If you experience adverse effects with a dose increase, drop the dose back down to the dose you were tolerating. Where possible, it may be ideal to use a liquid iron supplement to allow more flexibility in dosing. Iron supplementation may replenish iron stores more slowly at lower doses; however, it is more important that you feel good on any supplements you're taking. See the Additional Resources section or download your own copy here: https://resources. flourishingwithfibromyalgia.com/fibromyalgia-resource-guide for tips on starting new supplements with fibromyalgia.

In more extreme cases when an iron supplement is not tolerated at all, this may be due to low stomach acid levels (also known as hypochlorhydria). It may be necessary to address the low stomach acid levels prior to supplementing with iron. See Chapter 10 for more information on rebalancing the gut. If an iron supplement is not tolerated, increasing your intake of iron-rich food and cooking food in cast-iron pans can help increase iron stores and may be more tolerable than a supplement. See the Additional Resources section or download your own copy here: https://resources.flourishingwithfibromyalgia.com/ fibromyalgia-resource-guide for more information. Some health care providers can also administer iron injections. Speak with your health care provider about your options for iron replenishing.

## Vitamin B12 Deficiency

Vitamin B12 is easy to measure with blood testing and can result in a number of symptoms when deficient. Replenishing vitamin B12 is very easy and tends to be well tolerated. Vitamin B12 is widely available in animal-based foods, but if an individual is eating animal-based foods and is still deficient in vitamin B12, supplementation is necessary. There is additional evidence showing that supplementation with vitamin B12, even when there is no evidence of a deficiency, improves the symptoms of fibromyalgia patients.[60]

Vitamin B12 can be taken orally or administered as an injection. Oral supplementation with 1000mcg to 2000mcg of methylcobalamin daily, taken with food, can be used for three to six months to address a deficiency. Alternatively, injections are most commonly administered as 1000mcg or 5000mcg doses, and different forms of vitamin B12 may be used. Injection schedules for vitamin B12 can vary but may include weekly injections for four to six weeks, followed by a monthly injection for up to three months.[59] In research performed on people with fibromyalgia and myalgic encephalomyelitis, long-term weekly high-dose vitamin B12 injections paired with oral folic acid supplementation provided the most benefit in energy and pain levels.[60] There is no consensus on optimal lab values; however, there is minimal risk for high blood levels of vitamin B12.[61]

## Vitamin D Deficiency

Vitamin D is called either 25-hydroxycholecalciferol or 25-hydroxyvitamin D on lab reports. Optimal blood levels and supplemental doses of vitamin D are controversial. Vitamin D levels can be classified into several categories. Lab values less than 12ng/mL (30nmol/L) are considered deficient and could result in bone conditions. Lab values less than 20ng/mL (50nmol/L) are considered insufficient. Blood levels between 20ng/mL and 50ng/mL (50nmol/L to 125nmol/L) are considered adequate.[62] While 25-hydroxycholecalciferol levels above

20ng/mL (50nmol/L) indicate sufficiency, optimal levels of vitamin D are more likely to be closer to 50ng/mL (125nmol/L) and up.[59]

The minimal dose range of vitamin D to prevent insufficiency is 1000–4000IU of vitamin D3.[59] Doses of vitamin D to correct a deficiency can be much higher and may approach 10,000IU of vitamin D3.[59] It is very important to consult with a health care provider prior to taking large doses of vitamin D. Vitamin D is stored in the body and can have detrimental effects if toxic levels are reached. Doses of vitamin D can vary widely and should be determined depending on the initial lab result for 25-hydroxyvitamin D.

## IRRITABLE BOWEL SYNDROME

It is estimated that 25%–81% of patients with fibromyalgia also have irritable bowel syndrome (IBS).[63] IBS and fibromyalgia share many similarities. IBS has no definitive cause and like fibromyalgia, no abnormalities are detected on standard lab testing and imaging.[64] IBS is correlated with anxiety and depression as well as sleep abnormalities.[64]

Irritable bowel syndrome is typically diagnosed in teenagers and young adults in their 20s.[64] Symptoms occur intermittently and irregularly, with the condition flaring at different times and with different triggers.[64] Symptoms include abdominal discomfort or pain that feels like cramping and is often related to defecation. Abdominal discomfort may be related to changes in stool frequency (i.e., having a bowel movement more or less often) and changes in stool consistency (i.e., having looser or harder stools). Many patients experience alternation between constipation and diarrhea.[64] Overall, the experience of having a bowel movement is unpleasant for IBS sufferers. Many patients report straining, urgency, a feeling of incomplete bowel movements, mucus in the stool, and bloating with IBS.[64]

An official diagnosis of IBS is only given once all other possible causes have been ruled out.[64] This is called a diagnosis of exclusion. The Rome criteria were developed to categorize symptoms of IBS and standardize its diagnosis. To fit the Rome criteria, abdominal pain must be present for at least one day per week in the last three months, along with two or more of the following:[64]

- Pain related to defecation
- Pain associated with a change in frequency of defecation (i.e., having a bowel movement more or less often)
- Pain associated with a change in stool consistency (i.e., having looser or harder stools)

A number of physiologic abnormalities have been noted in people with IBS that may contribute to the symptoms. In people with IBS, there are abnormalities in how the intestines move, how sensitive the intestines are to different symptom triggers, and the amount of stretch the tissue tolerates.[64] A number of genetic and environmental factors have also been linked to the development of IBS, including differences in pathways connecting the gut and the brain, exposure to pathogenic bacteria, and certain medications.[64]

While controversial, it is estimated that up to 78% of IBS patients also have small intestinal bacterial overgrowth (SIBO).[65] Performing a glucose hydrogen breath test for SIBO is highly useful in cases of IBS, as the treatment for SIBO can differ significantly from the treatment for IBS.[65] As we will discuss later in this chapter, SIBO is highly correlated with fibromyalgia as well.

An entire book could be written on the treatment options available for IBS. While this book is written with the intention of treating fibromyalgia, many of the strategies discussed here apply to IBS treatment as well. In short, it is worthwhile to have a SIBO breath test done if that option is available to you. The most effective IBS treatment options I use in my practice are implementing a low-FODMAP diet, optimizing digestion, and managing stress. More information on these topics can be found in Chapters 6 and 7, as well as the Additional Resources section. Download your own copy of the Resource Guide here: https://resources.flourishingwithfibromyalgia.com/fibromyalgia-resource-guide

## MIGRAINES

Migraines are very severe headaches that can be debilitating, preventing the sufferer from functioning during an episode. Migraines are typically accompanied by pain in the head that is throbbing or pulsing in nature, but they can also occur without pain. If a migraine is experienced with pain, the pain typically occurs on one side of the head and may be accompanied by nausea and vomiting. Sensitivity to light, sound, or odours is also a common experience with migraines.[66]

Many migraine sufferers experience a prodrome before a migraine attack. A prodrome is a sensation that signals to the sufferer that a migraine is coming. Symptoms of a prodrome may include mood changes, loss of appetite, nausea, or other symptoms that consistently occur before a migraine. Auras may also occur before a migraine. Auras are disturbances in neurological function that may include changes in sensation, balance, muscle coordination, speech, or vision. Many also experience difficulty concentrating. Prodromes and auras can be short (lasting minutes) or can last up to one hour. Auras may last for the duration of the migraine or may occur without the sensation of pain.[66]

The pain of a migraine may last anywhere from a few hours to several days. Sufferers typically feel better with sleep and limited sensory stimulation, which may include limiting light, sound, and exposure to other people and activities. The frequency of migraine attacks varies widely from person to person.[66] Many women experience migraines at specific times in their menstrual cycle, while others cannot correlate their symptoms with their cycle. Most people can identify specific triggers that bring on a migraine. These triggers may include particular foods, skipping meals, stress, weather changes, sleep deprivation, neck pain, hormones, and exposure to specific stimuli (such as flashing lights).[66] It is estimated that up to 80% of people with fibromyalgia experience migraines.[67]

It is believed that migraines are caused by changes in blood flow within the brain along with inflammation in a number of nerves involved in the detection of pain within the brain.[66] Treatment for migraines should involve identifying triggers and minimizing exposure to them. This often starts with an elimination diet or food sensitivity test, as well as tracking the circumstances in which migraines occur with a migraine diary. Stress management and hormone balancing may also be included in the treatment plan, depending on what other triggers we are able to identify. There are a couple of simple tricks I use with patients to help abort a migraine if they feel one coming on. Some patients can consume caffeine (usually in the form of one to two cups of hot coffee) to prevent a full-blown migraine attack. Research on the effects of caffeine on migraines is mixed, but some people benefit when it is used acutely, whereas daily use can trigger migraines.[68] Other patients do better with a hydrotherapy technique that involves placing your feet in warm water while a cold, wet cloth is on the back of your neck. Please make sure you are seated while doing this, as it can make you dizzy. This technique draws blood flow away from the brain. I find that patients respond to either caffeine or hydrotherapy, but they are unlikely to respond to both. There are also a number of supplements that can be added to prevent and/or relieve migraines, most of which are discussed throughout this book in relation to fibromyalgia.

## RESTLESS LEG SYNDROME

Restless leg syndrome is a disorder involving an abnormal inclination to move the legs, arms, or other body parts. This urge to move often occurs along with abnormal sensations in the limbs, such as creeping or crawling sensations, or less commonly, pain in the extremities. Symptoms tend to worsen at night, when you are inactive or reclined. Because moving temporarily relieves the symptoms, many people with restless leg syndrome have difficulty falling asleep or wake frequently throughout the night.[69] The symptoms of restless leg syndrome are exacerbated by stress.

Research indicates that restless leg syndrome affects up to 65% of people with fibromyalgia. This is much higher than in the general population, where its incidence is estimated at up to 15%. Sleep quality is much lower when restless leg syndrome occurs alongside fibromyalgia, making symptoms of fibromyalgia worse.[70]

Restless leg syndrome can also occur due to drug withdrawal, as an adverse effect of medication, during pregnancy, and alongside a number of other conditions including kidney or liver failure, iron deficiency, anemia, diabetes, and neurologic disorders such as Parkinson's disease or multiple sclerosis.[69] Identifying which of these factors are contributing to the development of restless leg syndrome is important in determining how to treat the condition. If no identifiable cause can be found, supplementation with magnesium bisglycinate, performing limb stretches before bed, appropriate hydration, and managing stress are effective strategies to help relieve symptoms.

## DEPRESSION AND ANXIETY

Mood conditions are very common with fibromyalgia, and they may be present before the diagnosis of fibromyalgia is established or develop afterwards. Depression is more than just feeling sad. When experiencing depression, you may also feel tired, have difficulty concentrating, lose interest in doing things you used to enjoy, lose interest in sexual activity, and have difficulty sleeping or sleep more than normal. Some individuals experiencing depression may have thoughts of suicide or use substances to relieve the symptoms.[71] You may not be able to identify what is making you feel sad, but the feeling persists. There are a number of different diagnoses that may fit your symptoms if you are experiencing depression. In addition, certain physical conditions and nutrient deficiencies can result in symptoms of depression. To properly diagnose depression, these physical conditions must be investigated and ruled out as possible causes.

Depression and anxiety often occur together. As with depression, anxiety can fall into a number of different categories depending on when symptoms are experienced. For example, if social situations provoke anxiety, the diagnosis may be social phobia. If an individual is anxious or worries about a number of different activities or events, a diagnosis of generalized anxiety disorder may be more appropriate.[72] Other people with anxiety experience panic attacks. Although some worry is normal and healthy, anxiety becomes a problem when it disrupts your daily life and gets in the way of other feelings, such as happiness. Additional symptoms that can occur along with difficulty controlling worry include restlessness, feeling on-edge, getting tired easily, difficulty concentrating, irritability, muscle tension, and difficulty sleeping.[72]

Along with depression and anxiety, you may experience a feeling of loss for the life you used to have before fibromyalgia. My patient Gina had difficulty putting this feeling into words at first. She described it as feeling as though the "old her" had died, and she missed that part of herself. Gina felt a sense of grief over aspects of her life she had taken for granted before, like being able to get through a work day and go out with friends afterwards or running errands and being able to put away the groceries as soon as she got home without needing a nap. She described this feeling as being similar to mourning a loved one after they pass. It can be a difficult experience and one that not many people relate to.

When considering what the experience of having fibromyalgia is like, it seems obvious to me that depression and anxiety would be common. You're living in pain and constant discomfort with very little energy, frequently being told that there's nothing anyone can do, and you must be exaggerating. Very few people understand what you're going through because they can't see anything physically wrong with you. I think that's enough to make anyone feel sad and lonely. As the icing on the cake, you may not be able to work, see friends or family, or have much idea what your health will look like in the future. That's a lot of worry to carry.

There are many natural treatment options for depression and anxiety. Typically, once you find a treatment plan that is effective for your fibromyalgia symptoms, depression and anxiety symptoms improve as well. If your depression and anxiety are getting in the way of your motivation to start a plan to improve your health, treating these symptoms is a great place to begin. See Chapter 14 for details on natural treatments for depression and anxiety. Not every treatment option will be a good fit for your situation. A number of natural options interact with medications you may be on. Always check with your health care provider before starting a new supplement.

## SMALL INTESTINAL BACTERIAL OVERGROWTH (SIBO)

Small intestinal bacterial overgrowth (SIBO) is an overgrowth of bacteria in the small intestine.[73] Normally, most bacteria that live in the gut are present in the large intestine and colon. With SIBO, larger bacterial populations than expected live higher up in the intestines and can cause a variety of symptoms, including chronic diarrhea or constipation, bloating, abdominal pain or discomfort, flatulence, and weakness. Many people with SIBO also experience malabsorption of nutrients, unintentional weight loss, and nutrient deficiencies.[73]

SIBO is a relatively new condition and is much more common than previously thought.[73] Diagnosis of SIBO is still controversial; however, it is most commonly diagnosed using a breath test to measure the types and amounts of gases produced when a sugar solution is consumed.[65] The sugar solution usually consists of either glucose or lactose, with glucose showing more accurate results for diagnosing SIBO.[65] The results of this test can help guide treatment options. Common themes in the histories of patients with SIBO are frequent or long-term use of medications that lower stomach acid, frequent or long-term use of antibiotics, and a history of food poisoning. Some patients with SIBO feel worse when taking a probiotic. Treatment involves eradicating the dysbiotic bacteria, encouraging proper motility of the small intestine, and supporting healthy gut bacteria balance.

Research is just beginning to show that SIBO and fibromyalgia are strongly linked.[74] In research performed comparing hydrogen breath testing performed in people with IBS and people with fibromyalgia, a positive test result was more common with fibromyalgia than with IBS.[74] Other research performed on the populations of gut bacteria present in people with fibromyalgia has been able to link specific bacterial populations with the symptoms and severity of fibromyalgia.[33] It is difficult to estimate how many fibromyalgia patients also have SIBO without further research. If your digestive symptoms are resistant to most treatments, it may be worthwhile to be tested for SIBO.

## MYALGIC ENCEPHALOMYELITIS/ CHRONIC FATIGUE SYNDROME (ME/CFS)

Myalgic encephalomyelitis (formerly known as chronic fatigue syndrome) can be difficult to distinguish from fibromyalgia, and the conditions commonly occur together. ME is characterized by severe fatigue lasting at least six months that cannot be explained by any other diagnosis. Along with fatigue, many patients experience chronic swollen lymph nodes, low-grade fever, and frequent sore throats. The onset of ME is typically abrupt. It often follows an initial illness that resembles a viral infection, with symptoms such as fever, swollen lymph nodes, extreme fatigue, and upper respiratory symptoms. Unlike fibromyalgia, there is no prominent pain with ME, unless another co-occurring condition is present.

A number of infectious agents have been proposed as possible causes of ME, but none have been proven at this time. In studies investigating the immune systems of people with ME, a number of abnormalities have been identified. These abnormalities include low levels of several types of immune cells and poor functioning of other types of immune cells.[75] Natural treatment for ME involves immune-supportive therapies.

## MULTIPLE CHEMICAL SENSITIVITY (MCS)

Multiple chemical sensitivity (MCS) is also known as environmental illness or idiopathic environmental intolerance. This condition is poorly defined and poorly understood. People with MCS develop a number of symptoms when exposed to chemical substances via inhalation, touch, or ingestion, in the absence of organ dysfunction or physical signs. People with MCS have to be extremely careful about the environments they put themselves into, as they can end up very sick from the slightest exposure. Common triggers for MCS include alcohol and drugs, caffeine, food additives, carpet and furniture odours, fuel odours, engine exhaust, painting materials, perfume and scented products, pesticides, and herbicides.[76] Many people with MCS also report sensitivity to energy frequencies and wireless internet exposure.

It is estimated that approximately 16% of people with fibromyalgia also have MCS.[76] A large variety of symptoms can result from an exposure, including palpitations, chest pain, sweating, shortness of breath, fatigue, flushing, dizziness, choking, trembling, numbness, coughing, hoarseness, difficulty concentrating, and mood swings.[76] Diagnosis involves the elimination of other possible causes such as allergies, endocrine disorders, and building-related illnesses. Avoidance of exposure and support of the detoxification and elimination pathways in the liver and kidneys are the mainstay of natural treatment for MCS.

## KEY POINTS

- There are a number of conditions that commonly occur with fibromyalgia.
- These conditions may improve with fibromyalgia treatment, but they may also require treatment on their own.

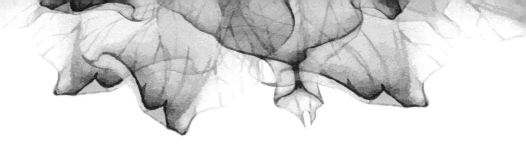

## SECTION 2

# The Essential Steps in Fibromyalgia Treatment

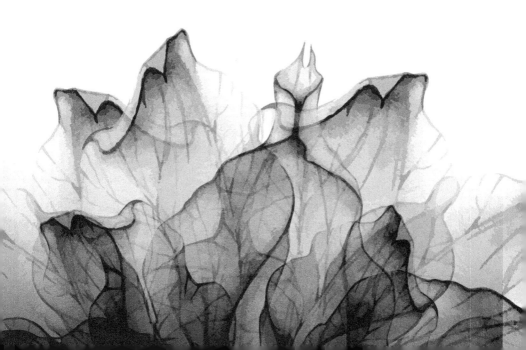

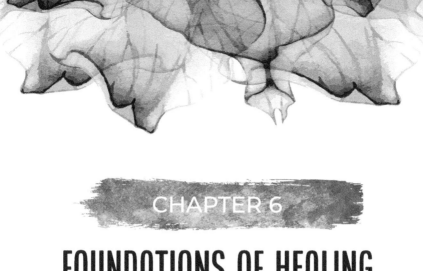

# CHAPTER 6

# FOUNDATIONS OF HEALING

Now that you know all about what fibromyalgia is and what other conditions commonly occur with it, it's time to jump into how to work on fixing the issues we've identified. The foundations of healing are important aspects of your life that affect your health in a profound way. You wouldn't build a house on a poor foundation, because anything you put on that foundation wouldn't hold up as well or as long. We need a strong foundation in place to build upon. The same goes for your health. If you are not sleeping well or digesting properly, no supplement we add will be as effective as it could be, resulting in lost time and money. Some of these aspects may seem incredibly basic, but I promise you they are worth your effort. When the foundations of healing are in place, many people experience significant improvements in their health, and they don't need to swallow another pill or spend more money to enjoy them. These basic lifestyle changes absolutely *must* be in place before you move on to the *Advanced Treatment* section of this book.

## SLEEP

### What Is Normal Sleep?

The amount of sleep needed can vary depending on the individual. It is generally recommended to get eight to ten hours of sleep each night. You should wake feeling rested and ready to take on the day. You should feel sleepy at your bedtime, and it should not take you more than 30 minutes to fall asleep. Ideally, I also like to hear that my patients dream most nights (whether they can remember it or not) and that they do not wake throughout the night most nights. If you experience nightmares, this can be a sign of stress, anxiety, or an adverse effect of sleep-inducing supplements or medications. Most adults should not have to wake during the night to go to the bathroom. See the *Sleep Hygiene* section in this chapter for tips on how to minimize nighttime awakening.

There are five stages in a normal sleep cycle. These stages can be measured by monitoring brain wave activity in a sleep study, called polysomnography. Stages 1 to 4 are called non-REM sleep and are considered lighter sleep. Stage 5 is the deepest stage of sleep, called REM sleep, which stands for rapid eye movement. Throughout the night, we cycle between non-REM and REM sleep.[77] In a normal sleep pattern, approximately 75%–80% of our total sleep time is spent in non-REM sleep, and 20%–25% of our total sleep time is spent in REM sleep. The first sleep cycle of the night is typically the shortest, lasting from 70–100 minutes. As the night progresses, the sleep cycle gets longer, lasting approximately 90–120 minutes, and the amount of time spent in REM sleep increases.[77] This means that as the night progresses, we spend more time in deeper sleep. REM sleep is when dreaming occurs.[77] Without a sleep study, we can determine that you are entering REM sleep throughout the night if you are dreaming. You may not be able to tell whether you dream every night, or you may not be able to recall your dreams, but this can be an indication of deeper sleep.

There are two hormones within the body that need to be in balance for proper restful sleep to occur. These hormones are melatonin and cortisol. Melatonin is the hormone associated with sleep. It is released in response to darkness and suppressed by exposure to light.[77] It is normally released at night to prepare the body for sleep.[77] Cortisol is termed the *stress hormone* and is responsible for the fight-or-flight response that protects us from danger. Cortisol is typically at its lowest levels during sleep and rises upon waking.[78] When stress levels are high, cortisol tends to reach higher levels, at least initially. Cortisol itself is not inherently bad. We do need it to function throughout the day and to protect us from danger. Cortisol can become a problem when we are exposed to chronically high levels, when we cannot bring cortisol levels down, or when we reach burnout and our body stops producing the cortisol we need or can no longer respond to it effectively.

## What Is Wrong with Sleep in People with Fibromyalgia?

Sleep studies performed on people with fibromyalgia have shown significant abnormalities in sleep patterns. Sleep abnormalities are estimated to affect up to 90% of people with fibromyalgia.[8] You may wake in the morning feeling as though you were awake most of the night, and you didn't get into a deep sleep. This is probably because that's exactly what happened.

Sleep studies in fibromyalgia have shown a shorter total sleep time, longer periods of waking after going to bed, and lighter sleep compared to people without fibromyalgia.[79] Although no specific sleep pattern has been identified as characteristic of fibromyalgia, abnormalities during specific stages of sleep have frequently been identified in people with fibromyalgia.[8,25] In sleep studies, people with fibromyalgia tend to spend less time in stages 3 and 4 of sleep, also known as slow-wave sleep. Some studies have also shown that people with fibromyalgia spend an increased percentage of total sleep time in stage 1, the lightest stage of sleep.[8] In addition to decreased time spent in stages 3 and 4, there are abnormalities in the types of brain waves we would expect to see in slow-wave sleep. This phenomenon is called alpha-wave intrusion, meaning that alpha waves intrude upon delta waves in sleep stages 3 and 4.[8,25] Alpha waves are brain waves present when the brain is in a relaxed state, such as during meditation. Delta waves are characteristic of deep, dreamless sleep. With alpha-wave intrusion, your brain is in a more wakeful state than normal during deeper sleep.[8]

In addition to the abnormalities we can measure in sleep studies, people with fibromyalgia report much difficulty with various aspects of sleep. Restlessness throughout the night, involuntary leg movements, feeling sleepy throughout the day, and an experience of non-refreshing sleep are common concerns in people with fibromyalgia.[8] People with fibromyalgia also report more difficulty falling asleep.[79] The compounded effect of lacking deep sleep and waking frequently means that you wake feeling tired and unrefreshed. When this happens night after night, it's no wonder you have trouble functioning because you're so tired.

You may also have noticed that after a particularly bad night, you not only feel extremely tired, but you are also in much more pain. Research has shown that the relationship between sleep quality and pain in people with fibromyalgia appears to go both ways. Poor sleep quality leads to increased pain, and high pain levels can also disrupt sleep.[8,28] Sleep is a time when the body does a ton of healing and rebalancing. Studies performed on the effects of sleep deprivation show adverse effects on the functioning of the cardiovascular, endocrine, immune, and nervous systems with chronic sleep times of less than seven hours per night. In addition, people who were sleep-deprived were more likely to suffer from anxiety and depression.[77] In fibromyalgia specifically, with poor sleep quality cognitive performance declines, and symptoms of fibro fog may be more prominent.[27] When we don't sleep well, every little task feels so much harder. It takes far more concentration and effort to get things done compared to when we feel well-rested. It's harder to manage our emotions, and we are much more easily frustrated.

So why is sleep so dysfunctional in fibromyalgia when you know that getting a good night's sleep is important? We've already discussed the evidence that points to brain inflammation and an abnormal stress response as possible contributors to fibromyalgia.[31] These two factors definitely play a role, but it's hard to say which came first. I highly suspect that a dysfunctional stress response comes before sleep dysfunction. Brain inflammation could either be a contributor to or a result of a lack of sleep. Regardless of how it came about, there are a number of strategies we can use to correct it, and it is the first, most important step in your journey to living well with fibromyalgia.

## Sleep Hygiene

Sleep hygiene is what we call the basic lifestyle practices and habits that need to be in place to support sleep. We will go through the most important practices here. I have included a detailed handout on sleep hygiene in the Additional Resources section. Download your own copy here: https://resources.flourishingwithfibromyalgia.com/fibromyalgia-resource-guide. The better you become at practicing sleep hygiene consistently, the more effective any supplements or herbs will be and the less likely you will be to require higher doses.

## Sleep Environment

The first aspect we target with sleep hygiene is sleep environment. This includes your bedroom and your bed itself. An ideal bedroom environment is quiet and cooler in temperature. It makes sense that you are going to lie awake if you are hearing lots of noises, such as other people in your household or traffic noise. Minimizing this as much as possible is ideal. It may be necessary to have conversations with other members of your household about quiet hours or moving more noisy activities (such as television) to rooms farther away from sleeping areas. Some noise may be unavoidable. If this is the case, placing a fan or white noise machine in the bedroom can help muffle other sounds. In regard to temperature, your body temperature naturally drops slightly when you sleep.[77] You know the wonderful feeling of being wrapped up and toasty warm in your blankets when the room itself feels a little colder? There's a physiologic basis to that feeling. When you are too warm during the night, you'll have a more restless sleep and wake more frequently. Dropping the temperature slightly at night, having a window open, or using lighter bedding can all help support sleep by encouraging this drop in body temperature.

As we've already discussed, exposure to light suppresses melatonin production. Turning off all lights and using blackout curtains or blinds can help encourage proper melatonin release and promote restful sleep. Opening the curtains and exposing yourself to sunlight upon waking for the day suppresses melatonin production and helps encourage balance between melatonin and cortisol levels. It may be helpful to use a night-light if you tend to wake at night to use the bathroom. If this is necessary, make sure the light is dim and is placed outside of the bedroom.

While light, noise, and temperature are all important, the most important rule about the bedroom is that it is used for sleep and intimacy only.

You should not be using your bedroom for work, homework, watching television, using the computer, or engaging in your hobbies. All of these activities need to be done outside of your bedroom. We need to retrain your body that the bedroom is a relaxing and sleepy environment. Removing any clutter, work-related materials, and unnecessary items from the bedroom will help encourage this connection in your brain.

Often, when I ask my patients about their bed itself, they haven't given it much thought. Your bed is absolutely essential to your ability to get restful sleep and minimize pain. Do you like your mattress? Do you find it comfortable? Do you know how old it is? How about your pillow? When was the last time you replaced it?

Mattresses can be a tricky subject. They can be expensive, and there may be some disagreement between partners who sleep together on which mattress they like best. There is no specific mattress that is best for people with fibromyalgia. It depends on what you prefer. I highly recommend shopping at a designated mattress store where staff are trained to help you find a mattress that works for you. Carve out enough time to shop for a new mattress, as it is recommended that you lay on a mattress for 15 minutes before determining whether you like it. If finances are a concern, be sure to shop during a sale. I know mattresses can be expensive, but so is taking supplements and medications long term. Mattresses should be replaced every seven to ten years, depending on their quality.

A good-quality pillow is also essential to your quest for restful sleep. Again, the best place to shop for a pillow is a mattress store. Good-quality pillows are designed to support your head and neck, depending on your sleep position. A pillow for someone who sleeps on their side should not look the same as a pillow for someone who sleeps on their back. Pillows should be replaced every six months to two years, again depending on the quality of the pillow. Many people with fibromyalgia notice a substantial difference in sleep quality, energy, and pain levels when they find the right mattress and pillow for them. I promise this is a worthwhile investment.

We've already touched upon bedding, but it is also very important for sleep. Bedding should be light enough that you are not overheating or sweating during the night, but heavy enough that you are not feeling cold. It should be made of a comfortable material. The same goes for pyjamas, if you wear them. Many people sleep better in the nude. I recommend that you do whatever you feel comfortable with and what works for your lifestyle.

*Bedtime Routine*

Besides sleep environment, bedtime routine is the area I find we can make the most improvements in to support sleep. Implementing these tips may require some planning and shuffling of your evening routine, but they are worthwhile. With respect to bedtime routine, we are generally talking about the one-hour time period before you go to bed and the act of going to bed itself.

Let's work backwards. What time should you be going to bed? In an ideal world, between 10p.m. and 11p.m. is the best time to go to bed based on how your cortisol and melatonin circadian rhythm works. Most of the time, the people I see with fibromyalgia have bedtimes much later than this (in the 1a.m. to 4a.m. range). I understand how this happens. When sleep is challenging, you start to dread going to bed. You associate the whole bedtime process with frustration and anxiety. Despite your best efforts, you still can't sleep the way you'd like to, so why bother trying? We're going to get you back on track and sleeping well, and it will happen overnight, though maybe not on the first night.

So, if your bedtime is much later than 10p.m., how do you make your body go to bed at 10p.m.? We gradually train your body to go to bed earlier. The first step is to determine what your starting bedtime is. You may decide this is what time you climb into bed, but in reality, your bedtime is shortly before the time you get sleepy and your body is ready for rest. Lying awake in bed for hours is common with fibromyalgia, and this is the pattern we want to break, as it trains your body that the bed is not necessarily associated with sleep. If you are going to bed at 12a.m. but not falling asleep until 2a.m., then your starting bedtime is 1:30a.m. (about 30 minutes before you fall asleep).

If your starting bedtime is 1:30a.m., and we want to work towards an earlier bedtime, we will first push your bedtime earlier by 30 minutes to a new bedtime of 1:00a.m. You stick with this new bedtime of 1:00a.m. until you are consistently falling asleep by 1:30a.m. at the latest. I generally find it takes about two weeks to adjust to a new bedtime. Once you are consistently falling asleep at your new bedtime, we push your bedtime earlier by another 30 minutes (to 12:30a.m. in our example). This process continues until you are consistently falling asleep at a time closer to 10:00 p.m., without lying awake in bed for hours. I know this process sounds long, but it will be much less frustrating than trying to go to bed at 10:00 p.m. right from the start. Your body will not adjust to that routine very easily or quickly, and you will be more likely to give up on adjusting your bedtime.

It is normal to have the odd night when you don't fall asleep until later. As we'll discuss in the *Energy Conservation* section of this chapter, this is often because of the events of the day and taking on too much. If your sleep schedule is very sporadic, your first step may be to implement a consistent routine before pushing towards an earlier bedtime.

Once you've determined what your bedtime is, you will know when the one hour before your bedtime falls. This one-hour time period is what we consider the time dedicated to your *bedtime routine*. This hour is used to prepare you for bed and signals to your body that it is almost time for sleep. If necessary, you can set an alarm 15 minutes before your bedtime routine is to begin (1 hour and 15 minutes before bedtime) to signal that you are to finish up whatever task you are engaged in and start your bedtime routine. Your bedtime routine includes all of the normal things you do before bed, such as brushing your teeth, washing your face, putting on your pyjamas, etc. This time also includes relaxing and unwinding. Most people would include watching TV or playing on their phone as relaxing and unwinding. The caveat here is that this one-hour period is a screen-free period. As we discussed above, light, especially blue light from electronic devices, suppresses melatonin release and will disrupt sleep. Most people will argue that they have a blue light filter on their phone or computer. In my opinion, sleep is absolutely essential to your health and improvement, so I recommend that you have a screen-free hour before bed. Schedule some time to spend on your phone or computer before your one-hour bedtime routine.

It is also best to avoid eating or drinking during the one-hour bedtime routine period. Avoid drinking shortly before bed to help prevent you from waking during the night to go to the bathroom. Digesting food can also disrupt your sleep and is not ideal. The exception to this rule is if you tend to wake in the night a few hours after falling asleep and are not sure why, as in, you're not physically uncomfortable, worrying, or needing to go to the bathroom. If you are waking shortly after falling asleep and are not sure why, this can be a sign that your blood sugars are dropping, which could cause you to wake up. Adding in a bedtime snack within the one hour before bedtime, containing both protein and natural sugars, can help prevent this. Examples of a great bedtime snack include fruit and nut butter or fruit and cheese, depending on your dietary preferences. The best way to determine if this will help your sleep is to give it a try for a few nights.

Beyond avoiding screens, eating or drinking, and working in the one hour before bed, you can use this time however you like, as long as it's relaxing and you're getting to bed at your scheduled bedtime. Many people use this time to read or engage in a hobby that they find relaxing. This one-hour period is a great time to meditate and work on calming the body's stress response. We will discuss meditation later on in this chapter. I know these changes may seem very different from what you're doing now, but that's the point. What you're doing now clearly isn't working for you, so give these changes a try and see how much your sleep can improve with just the basics.

## Sleep Apnea

I see a number of patients with both fibromyalgia and sleep apnea. The treatment of sleep apnea is beyond the scope of this book. If you have a breathing-assistance machine for the treatment of sleep apnea, it is important that you use it and use it properly. Sleep hygiene and natural treatments for improving sleep will not be as effective if you have untreated sleep apnea. Untreated sleep apnea also makes the symptoms of fibromyalgia much worse and can be a huge barrier to improvement.

## DIGESTION

Digestion is the second foundation of healing we will discuss in this chapter. There are few things we do more often than sleeping and eating. That is why these two foundations are so important for our overall well-being. Digestion and diet have the power to make us healthy or make us very ill. In this section, we will discuss how to ensure your digestive system is functioning optimally. Dietary strategies will be discussed in Chapter 7.

As discussed in Chapter 5, there are several digestive conditions that commonly occur alongside fibromyalgia, including irritable bowel syndrome (IBS) and small intestinal bacterial overgrowth (SIBO). The specific treatments pertaining to these conditions are outside the scope of this book; however, many of the following strategies related to digestion and diet will help improve these conditions, as well as fibromyalgia symptoms. If you suspect you have SIBO (or SIBO that is misdiagnosed as IBS), I recommend you seek advice from a health care provider with experience treating SIBO. Treatment protocols can be long and involved, but the outcomes are very often worthwhile.

## Mindful Eating

Our society and the way we live our daily lives have wreaked havoc on our digestive systems, which is why we're starting with the basics of how to support our digestive systems from a lifestyle perspective. We live in a world where it is considered desirable to be on-the-go at all times and have every minute of every day scheduled. We have moved away from sitting down at the dinner table to eat our meals, in favour of eating while working, driving, or skipping meals altogether. We are all guilty of this to some extent, but our bodies do not fare well with this style of eating, and practicing the guidelines here will be an important aspect of your journey to a healthy digestive system and living well with fibromyalgia.

We have two nervous systems within our bodies with very different functions. The first is the parasympathetic nervous system, which is responsible for *rest-and-digest* functions. The second is the sympathetic nervous system, which is responsible for *fight-or-flight* functions. The sympathetic nervous system is responsible for ensuring we react appropriately when faced with danger, either by fighting the attacker or by running away from the source of danger. The parasympathetic nervous system helps to calm us down and is responsible for sleep and digestion. These two nervous systems cannot be active at the same time. You are either in rest-and-digest mode, or you are in fight-or-flight mode, with energy and resources directed appropriately. This means that when we are living our busy, stressful lives (in fight-or-flight mode), we cannot appropriately direct the energy and resources necessary for resting and digesting.

This is where mindful eating comes in. Mindful eating is the practice of paying attention to what you eat and how you eat it. The practice of mindful eating involves stopping what you are doing to engage in the act of eating, taking the time to taste your food and chew it properly, and eating regularly throughout the day. While this all sounds easy, we as a society seem to have difficulty practicing these principles, which adds stress to our already taxed digestive systems.

Mindful eating is particularly important in fibromyalgia. As we discussed in Chapter 2, people with fibromyalgia have developed an abnormal stress response over time. This means that your body is so used to being in fight-or-flight mode that it has trouble shifting into rest-and-digest mode when it needs to. You may not be eating on the run or skipping meals, but your body is responding as if you were. We need to calm your body so that you can switch into rest-and-digest mode more often. This will take practice, but the benefits will be well worth the effort.

### Step 1: Eat Regularly.

The first step to mindful eating is to ensure that you are eating regularly throughout the day. Irregular eating habits trigger the starvation response and are an added stress that your body does not need. Irregular eating is also a common cause of low energy and energy crashes in people with fibromyalgia. I generally recommend three meals per day with one to three snacks, depending on your appetite level and the size of your meals. You may have heard that breakfast is the most important meal of the day. I think all meals are equally important, but breakfast is the meal that is most often skipped. When you skip breakfast, your body does not get the signal (food coming in) to get your metabolism going, and you continue in the fasting state that you were in overnight. Your brain and body do not operate as well in the fasting state. In this state, your body and brain are working to conserve as much energy as possible, since they have no idea how long the fast will last. You likely don't notice this when you're sleeping, but it can become more of a difficulty when you are awake and trying to function. We will discuss food choice in Chapter 7, as it is also very important in ensuring you are functioning at your best.

When I suggest eating three meals plus one to three snacks per day, many people say they don't have the appetite to eat that much. Listening to your body is very important, but you may have lost touch with your hunger cues if you have been eating irregularly for a long period of time. We may need to work on retraining your body to send hunger cues at the appropriate times (shortly after you wake up, for example). To do this, all you need to do is consume a small amount of food at times that would constitute a regular mealtime. For example, if you don't have an appetite for breakfast, try having a couple of bites of a banana with nut butter each morning when you wake up (you're aiming to consume some protein, but it doesn't have to be this example).

This will help train your body that it should expect some form of breakfast. If you can't eat large quantities, that is fine. Our goal is to shift your body and metabolism into a wakeful state, not necessarily to be prepared for a buffet breakfast. The other reason you may not have an appetite is poor digestive function, which we will discuss in more detail in Chapter 10.

*Step 2: Eat Slowly.*

Your brain and digestive system are communicating constantly, but it takes about 15 minutes for your brain to process that you are full. It also takes some time for your digestive organs to get the message to release the acid, digestive enzymes, and bile necessary to digest the food you've consumed. We tend to eat much too quickly, allowing partially digested food to pass through our digestive tracts and become food for the bacteria in our large intestines. While it's important that these bacteria are supported, they will get enough food from a healthy diet, without poor digestion allowing more undigested food to pass through.

When you are eating, it is important to sit down at a table with no screens (TVs, laptops, or cell phones) or distractions (work, homework, etc.). You should focus solely on eating and enjoying the different flavours on your plate. It is ideal to chew each bite of food about 30 times, as digestion begins in your mouth. I don't recommend you count how many times you've chewed a specific bite, but the food should be soft and have minimal flavour left once chewed thoroughly.

If you are particularly stressed or want to ensure you have entered into rest-and-digest prior to sitting down to eat, a great practice is to engage in a short meditation or deep breathing exercise before starting to eat. This practice works wonderfully in supporting digestion without the addition of another supplement or medication. We will discuss meditation further in the *Meditation* section of this chapter.

*Step 3: Choose Your Foods Mindfully.*

I often find that once we have discussed mindful eating, and my patients are paying more attention to what they are eating and how they are eating it, they realize how much flavour unseasoned food has. Since they are eating more slowly, they tend to avoid overeating and feel much better after a meal. Symptoms that can be decreased by practicing mindful eating alone include nausea, bloating, heartburn, stomach upset, and excessive fullness.

Mindful eating also involves choosing your food mindfully. We will discuss food choice more specifically in Chapter 7, but I want to go over the basics here. The general guideline that I recommend my patients follow when making a meal is to divide their plate into quarters. Ideally, we want half of the plate (two quarters) to be colourful vegetables (green, red, orange, purple, etc.). This can be one vegetable dish or two, depending on your preference. One quarter of your plate should be a protein source. This can either be a meat source of protein or a plant source (see the Additional Resources section or download your own copy here: https://resources.flourishingwithfibromyalgia. com/fibromyalgia-resource-guide, for more information on protein sources). The last quarter of your plate should be a carbohydrate source, preferably one that is minimally processed. Examples of this could include brown rice, quinoa, potatoes, beans, or lentils. Obviously, you will have meals that mix these different types of food, but approximately the same proportions should apply. As for treats, I recommend my patients have one treat meal or snack per week. This can take some time to work towards if you have a sweet or salty tooth, but if you gradually cut down, you can get there. I recommend that my patients choose this treat carefully and make sure they fully enjoy it (i.e., eat it mindfully). Avoiding large quantities of fluids with meals can also help improve digestion. Consuming lots of fluids right before or along with a meal dilutes your digestive juices and does not allow them to act as effectively. It is fine to sip a drink while eating but try to consume most of your fluids apart from meals by at least 30 minutes.

The effects of practicing mindful eating can be substantial. My patient Whitney came to see me with very low energy levels, lots of bloating, gas, and frequent nausea. She was not eating frequently because she felt awful every time she did eat. We discussed her diet and her eating habits. Whitney was used to being busy and on-the-go all the time, frequently forgetting to eat and eating very sporadically. We discussed the importance of food choices and taking the time to sit down and eat, rather than eating when distracted. I recommended that Whitney eat three meals per day and sit down at the table for 30 minutes each time she ate a meal. I also recommended she have an afternoon snack consisting of fruit and nuts. I instructed Whitney to pay more attention to what she was eating and to ensure she tasted her food. She was to practice eating with her opposite hand to slow down her food intake. Whitney was skeptical but willing to give it a try. When I saw Whitney two weeks later, she couldn't believe how much those small changes had improved her energy and digestion. Her energy level increased by 30%, and she wasn't crashing during the afternoon as often. By slowing down the speed of her eating, she was no longer feeling nauseous, and her bloating had also decreased substantially. Whitney was still finding it difficult to eat with her opposite hand, but by eating mindfully she learned how much she enjoyed eating a variety of vegetables. Mindful eating was just the beginning for Whitney and an important first step in allowing the digestive system to work optimally.

## ENERGY CONSERVATION

Do you know what a crash is? A crash occurs when you overextend yourself on an average or good day. That is, you weren't having a bad day, so you pushed yourself to do more than you normally would. Maybe you caught up on laundry or cleaned the entire house or attended a social event. By the end of the day you were exhausted. You would think that because you were exhausted you would sleep well, but you didn't. It was the worst sleep you've had in a while, and the next day you struggled to get out of bed. You felt even more exhausted, and you were in even more pain. You got even less done than you normally would.

Remember in Chapter 2 when we discussed the mitochondria? As a refresher, mitochondria are the parts of our cells that create energy in the form of a molecule called ATP. People with fibromyalgia have fewer mitochondria and defects in key enzymes, as well as nutrient deficiencies that contribute to dysfunctional energy production in mitochondria.[11,14-16] This means that they don't produce or regenerate ATP as efficiently as they should. This is why energy conservation is so important. Until we can correct the functioning of your mitochondria, we need to work on conserving the energy you do have so that you can function in your daily life and put in the required effort to work on your health. I like to use the analogy of making a deposit into your *energy piggy bank*. You're working hard on improving your overall energy level with the strategies outlined in this book (these are your deposits). You're doing this by making sure you are sleeping well, eating nutritious food, and supporting your mitochondria. To grow your *energy piggy bank*, you not only need to make regular deposits, but you also need to make sure that what you deposit stays in the piggy bank. If you take out as much as you deposit, you're going to stay in the same place, and you won't progress. By conserving your energy deposits, your energy level will improve over time.

Throughout your journey to living well with fibromyalgia, it will be important to learn to conserve the energy you have, so you don't end up in these crash cycles and stay bedridden for days. This practice is called *pacing* and it's a difficult one. It will take practice and self-discipline to prevent yourself from pushing your limits and instead conserving some of the energy you have worked so hard to build up.

Pacing involves working within the limits of the energy you have that day and finding ways to save energy where you can. Dr. Bested developed a tool called the Activity Log and Functional Capacity Scale that is used to track energy levels, activities throughout the day, and ability to function.[80] This is the tool we will use when practicing pacing. You can find a summary of the pacing directions in the *Additional Resources* section for later reference.

## Step 1: Record Your Hours of Sleep and Sleep Quality.

Under the day you are starting your activity log, record the number of hours you slept and the quality of your sleep on a scale of 1 to 5, with 1 being very poor and 5 being very good sleep.

## Step 2: Rate Your Energy at the Beginning of the Day.

At the start of your day, rate your energy on a scale of 0 to 10, based on where you fit on the functional capacity scale included with the activity log.[80] Record this before you do anything else.

## Step 3: Adjust the Times on the Left-Hand Side to Fit Your Schedule.

If you normally wake around 10a.m., adjust the times on the side accordingly, starting with 10a.m. Each time slot represents an hour of your day.

## Step 4: Record Your Activities and Functional Capacity Scale Rating throughout the Day.

The first few times you fill out the activity log, you may want to record your activities as you go and see how your functional capacity scale rating changes throughout the day. Later on, you can use the activity log to schedule your day and ensure you aren't pushing yourself beyond your limits. Every hour, record your activity and what your functional capacity scale rating is at that time. For example, in the 12p.m. slot you may write:

Ate lunch – 20 mins
Rest – 20 mins
Cleaned up – 20 mins
Functional Capacity Scale Rating = 3

You can develop your own short form to make filling out the activity log faster (for example, write "R" for rest and "C" for cleaning). I highly recommend recording your activities and functional capacity ratings as you go. If you try to record it all at the end of the day, you will not be able to remember how you were feeling in the moment.

## Step 5: Record the Number of Minutes You Exercised and the Number of Useable Hours in the Day.

Record the number of minutes you walked or exercised and the number of usable hours in the day. The useable hours in a day are hours when you are not asleep or resting with eyes closed.[80] While these numbers can be difficult to see at first, they are your starting point. It will be encouraging when you see these numbers go up and know you're on the right path.

## Step 6: Record Your Functional Capacity Scale Rating at the End of the Day.

Just before going to bed, record how you're feeling based on the functional capacity scale. Over time, we want to work on keeping your functional capacity rating consistent and prevent it from decreasing throughout the day.

## Step 7: Use Your Activity Log Daily.

Over time, you will be able to see patterns of when you pushed yourself too far and ended up with lower functional capacity ratings for the following days. You can start to identify where your limits are and how to work with them. You may even be able to identify which tasks are too much for you and work on strategies around them, either by asking for help with those tasks or by breaking them up into smaller chunks. You'll begin to see how important sleep is and how much it affects your ability to function the next day.

To help with identifying crashes and limits, it can be useful to colour-code your activity logs. For example, colouring low-energy times with red (rated as 0 to 3 on the functional capacity scale), moderate-energy times with yellow (rated as 4 to 7 on the scale), and high-energy times with green (rated as 8 to 10 on the scale) may provide a striking visual of how you're doing and where you can improve.

## Step 8: Use Your Activity Log to Schedule Your Day.

After completing a few activity logs, it's likely that you will be able to identify where you're overexerting yourself and ending up with lower functional capacity ratings at the end of the day. Ideally, we want you to start and end the day with around the same functional capacity rating. I know that sounds crazy, since what you really want is to be improving. The improvements will come over time, but to start with we want to conserve the energy you have. This concept is similar to saving your allowance, rather than blowing it all as soon as you get it. Over time, you will notice an upward trend in your functional capacity ratings if you're working within your limits during the day and implementing the other strategies in this book.

Using the activity logs you've already completed, you'll want to try to balance your day based on your functional capacity ratings. Some people find they can do more in the morning and then need to rest more in the afternoon and evening, or vice versa. If you function better in the morning, schedule your more challenging tasks in the morning and less energy-intensive tasks in the afternoon. Make sure you are scheduling rest periods throughout the day to recover from the tasks you are performing and maintain your functional capacity rating. Rest means that you are lying down with your eyes closed or sleeping. Activities such as watching TV or reading are low-energy activities, not rest. Rest periods don't necessarily have to be long but may need to be frequent. Find what works for you so that you can maintain the energy gains you will achieve. For tips and tricks on saving energy where possible, see the *Additional Resources* section.

## Warning about Activity Logs

Activity logs can be emotionally triggering at first. It can be very difficult to see how little you're accomplishing in a day. I encourage you to stick with it. As you make improvements, compare your activity logs from when you began, or when you were in a crash, to how you feel when you are doing well. This will be proof that when you take care of yourself, you can make improvements in your health, and will provide encouragement to keep working on it.

## MINDSET

The mindset we have plays a huge role in our health, our beliefs about our conditions, and what we are able to achieve. I believe this is one of the biggest barriers we need to overcome in getting you to a place where you feel you are living well with fibromyalgia. Before your fibromyalgia symptoms took over, you were the person who took care of everything. You were the person everyone came to for help, knowing that you wouldn't say no and they could count on you. You always did your best, and people noticed. You were great at your job, your friends and family loved spending time with you, and you were talented in your hobbies. Now your symptoms get in the way of your ambition, determination, and ability to help those around you. This is a big blow to your self-esteem. To top it off, you're being told by doctors, friends, family, and the media that you are never going to get better. That's a lot of negativity to contend with.

Let me be the first to tell you that I know you can get better. I know you can live the life you've always dreamed of, and I strongly believe that the world needs you. However, it's not enough for me to tell you. You need to believe it yourself. You need to believe that the work you're going to put into getting better will pay off, and you will be able to live your life the way you want to. I encourage you to continue to dream about what "one day" looks like and what you will do once your symptoms are not stopping you.

I understand that there is a lot of emotional processing and grief around being diagnosed with a condition like fibromyalgia. There's a lot of stigma and lots of unknowns about what your life and health will look like with fibromyalgia. I encourage you to identify with your diagnosis, but I caution you against letting it define you. You existed before you were diagnosed with fibromyalgia, and although it may have changed your life significantly, it will not ruin you so long as you don't let it.

How do you go about changing your mindset? It will happen in baby steps every day. It will require patience with yourself and dedication to short daily practices to shift your thoughts. I've included a couple of exercises for you to try. I encourage you to find ones that work for you and if you're willing, to work with a mental health professional to help you shift into a healthier mindset. I've included a summary of these exercises in the Additional Resources section and the downloadable Resource Guide (https://resources.flourishingwithfibromyalgia.com/ fibromyalgia-resource-guide) for your reference.

## Visualizations

To start, I want you to think about what your life would look like if you'd never been diagnosed with fibromyalgia, better yet if you'd never heard of it. What would you have accomplished? What would you have done differently? Who would you be spending your free time with? Are there any activities or hobbies you have given up that you wish you had continued? I want you to put this life into pictures or words (whichever works better for you). This is your *One Day Visualization*.

Next, I want you to identify a small part of your *One Day Visualization* that you want to work towards within the next six months. Recovery looks different for everyone, so timelines are flexible. For example, say you want to be able to go to the movie theatre and enjoy a whole film without crashing the next day or coming home feeling awful. That will be your six-month goal. Every time you're working on something for your health, whether it is taking your supplements, eating a stricter diet than you're used to, or pacing your activities and it's starting to feel like too much, remember your six-month goal. Baby steps will get you there, and it will feel so good when you've reached it.

When I started working with Taylor, we discussed goals and the importance of visualizing what she wanted to achieve if her symptoms weren't stopping her. She told me how much she used to love going to the movies. She was in so much pain and felt so tired that she couldn't make it through a whole movie without having to lie in bed for two days afterwards. It got to the point where she didn't even enjoy going to the movies anymore, because the crash afterwards wasn't worth it. Taylor put going to a movie on her *One Day Visualization*, and this was her six-month goal. Every time Taylor was having a bad day and feeling frustrated about her health journey, she reminded herself how badly she wanted to go to a movie and enjoy it. This helped her work extra hard at implementing the diet and lifestyle changes and remembering to take her supplements. I was scheduled to see Taylor at the six-month mark, but I got a call from her two weeks before our visit. She couldn't wait until the six-month mark and had gone to a movie over the weekend. She happily reported that she enjoyed every minute of it and could function the next day! We both did our happy dances and at our next visit, discussed adjusting the *One Day Visualization* to Taylor's next goal.

The point of this activity is not to discourage you, although I know it can feel that way when you're thinking of all of the things you can't do now. The idea is to give you points of reference for your journey to health. These are what you're working towards, and they will be your points of celebration once you get there. There will also be many small points of celebration, but these will be your big ones. These are the ones that will keep you going when it's beginning to feel like too much work. Pull out your *One Day Visualization* and remind yourself how much you deserve that life.

## Positive Affirmations

Negative self-talk is very common and can be incredibly emotionally draining. It can rob you of any motivation you once had to get better when that little voice inside your head keeps telling you that "you can't do it," "it's too hard," and "you're not worth it." Whether you've internalized this self-talk from abuse in your past or you're unsure where it came from, it's not serving you, and it's time to get rid of it.

Positive affirmations are a great way to drown out that negative voice. The more often you combat that negative voice with positive alternatives, the more likely you are to believe the positive thoughts. Doing positive affirmations and engaging in self-love can feel unnatural at first. If this is the case for you, I recommend framing your positive affirmations as phrases you would tell someone dear to you, whether it's your best friend, your child, or your significant other. A common positive affirmation I hear people use is "I am enough." While you are definitely enough, I wouldn't tell my best friend that she is enough. That just doesn't sound good enough for her. I would tell her something like, "you deserve everything you've ever wanted in life and more," or "you deserve to be loved unconditionally and treated like a queen." Find a phrase that works for you and use it. Say it out loud, repeat it in your head, put it on your mirror, or read it before you go to bed. Consistency is key with a positive affirmation practice.

If the first method still feels like too much for you, a simple reminder to your body and your mind of "I am safe" can bring a state of calm. Remember how we discussed the abnormal stress response in fibromyalgia and how we need to train your body to respond properly to stress? Your body forgets that it is, in this moment, safe. You may need to remind it when you're feeling stressed or anxious. Although you have worries and stresses, you are not in immediate danger, and you are safe.

## Meditation and Deep Breathing

Meditation and deep breathing are important exercises for calming that overactive stress response. Many people dislike meditating and find it difficult. There's a reason it's difficult. You're stuck in a stress response, and your body has forgotten how to relax. The more you practice getting your body into a relaxed state, the more often your body will default there, and the easier it will be to calm down when you're feeling stressed.

The other reason many of us find meditating difficult and don't bother with it is that when we think about meditating, we picture a Buddhist monk who sits in silence for hours. At least, that's what I used to picture. We do not need to meditate for hours. We don't even need to fully prevent our minds from wandering while we meditate in order to benefit from it.

When I recommend meditation to my patients, I suggest that they start with just two minutes per day. Most people fit this in before bedtime or first thing in the morning. Regardless of when you do it, you have two minutes per day to spare. What you do in this two-minute time frame is mostly up to you, as long as you find the practice relaxing and engage in it fully. You can do deep breathing, listen to a guided meditation, or pray. A guided meditation doesn't have to be a recording telling you when to breathe. It could be a visualization of a walk through a forest or along a beach. Find a meditation that works for you and use it. I've included some options in the *Additional Resources* section that you can use to guide your meditation time.

## EXERCISE

If you can't exercise right off the bat, don't let it stress you. I include the exercise section here because it is a lifestyle component of your journey that you will want to implement when you can. When we speak of exercise, we're not talking about spending an hour or more at the gym doing cardio and resistance training. We're talking about getting the body moving. Period. However that works for you. Research has shown that people with fibromyalgia experience fewer symptoms when they exercise regularly, but you are the expert on your body and know it best.[1] If now is not the time, we'll make progress in other aspects of your health and revisit exercise later.

There are a number of reasons why exercise is important in fibromyalgia. First, exercise encourages blood flow. If you recall from Chapter 2, muscle biopsies in people with fibromyalgia showed that there was not enough blood flow to the tissues.[11,13] Blood brings nutrients and oxygen to tissues and cleans out waste products. Without adequate blood flow, tissues do not have the nutrients necessary to grow and repair themselves. They also accumulate waste products, which can be toxic. Appropriate blood flow is important for all tissues in the body, including the brain and muscles. The second reason is that exercise is very beneficial for joints. Our joints have fluid within them that allows the different body parts to move over each other smoothly and without damage. When we move, this fluid is replenished with fresh fluid full of nutrients. Exercise also has a huge variety of other benefits, including benefits for mood, concentration, digestion, strength, and metabolic efficiency. The key is to exercise within your tolerance and to introduce an exercise program slowly.

## Yoga

A number of research articles have been published on the use of yoga in people with fibromyalgia. These studies show that there may be some improvement in pain, fatigue, mood, and sleep with the practice of yoga in people with fibromyalgia.[81-83] Yoga may also be helpful in reducing stress, improving self-confidence, and addressing abnormalities in cortisol levels associated with fibromyalgia.[83-84] Not all studies show significant benefit; however, studies to date have been small and have included different forms of yoga. Yoga may be more beneficial with more consistent practice, as research has shown that participants who engaged in a daily at-home practice ranging from 25–40 minutes experienced the most benefit.[81-82]

Clinically, yoga is one of the forms of exercise I find my patients tolerate best. Practices don't necessarily need to be long, but can be significantly helpful in reducing pain levels, brain fog, and fatigue. I recommend you choose a form of yoga that is slow-moving, incorporates meditation or breathing exercises, and can be done at home. Yoga is great for stretching out tense muscles, encouraging blood flow around the body, and moving joints. I would highly discourage you from doing hot yoga or from attending an advanced class before seeing how you tolerate this at home. A beginner's class could be a great option if you find you are more likely to be successful in a group setting or with an instructor. I've included some great yoga resources in the *Additional Resources* section.

## Stretching

Whether you're engaging in a yoga practice or a whole-body stretching routine, your body will thank you. Stretching is easy to do in bed or when sitting and can be done relatively quickly. Starting a stretching routine can be a great way to begin a regular exercise practice and should always be incorporated at the end of a more advanced exercise program.

When stretching, it is ideal to feel the stretch, but not to stretch to the point of pain. You should hold a stretch for 20–30 seconds and stretch a particular muscle two or three times prior to moving on. Again, if this is too much for you, work within your limits. I've included resources you can access online in the *Additional Resources* section.

## Walking

Walking can be a great way to introduce exercise into your daily life. Walking, particularly outside, gives an instant mood boost. Be sure to start slowly and account for the time it will take you to get back. If you can, go with a friend or family member and have a plan for if you go too far. If you're working on increasing your walking time, be sure you are increasing it slowly. With all exercise, using the 10% rule is helpful. When you're feeling comfortable with the amount of time you're walking, and you don't experience any increase in symptoms as a result of exercise over a two-week period, increase the amount of time you walk by 10%. For example, if you're walking for 10 minutes every day, increase your daily walking time to 11 minutes (1 minute is 10% of 10 minutes).

## Swimming

Swimming is a great exercise option for people in pain, especially joint pain. When you are in the water, you do not have to hold up your own body weight and can move more freely. In fibromyalgia, aquatic exercise shows benefit in improving overall well-being, ability to perform daily activities, stiffness, and fitness.[85] There has been no consensus on what forms of aquatic exercise are best for fibromyalgia, and it is unclear whether the benefit may be partially due to the temperature of the water.[85]

My patient Yvonne had been a competitive swimmer as a teenager. When she was diagnosed with fibromyalgia at the age of 23, she had already given up swimming because she was too sore and tired afterwards. She couldn't recover like she used to. When I met Yvonne 17 years after her diagnosis, beginning to swim again wasn't on her to-do list. She just wanted to get the pain under control and live comfortably. Yvonne committed to a strict elimination diet to identify food triggers, practiced sleep hygiene and pacing, and we added supplements to support her sleep and mitochondrial function. We planned to add exercise once she was feeling better. Four months after our initial visit together, Yvonne was thrilled to be swimming twice per week. With further progress in her pain and energy, she was looking to start teaching swimming lessons. Swimming provided Yvonne with some much-needed movement to relieve the soreness in her muscles and joints.

You don't need to be a competitive swimmer to start swimming. Swimming can be a tiring exercise, so make sure you start slowly and have a companion with you. Until you know how you tolerate swimming, stay in the shallow areas and take it slow. Where possible, choose to swim in pools with a warmer temperature.

## KEY POINTS

- Abnormal sleep in fibromyalgia can contribute to more severe pain and cognitive difficulties.
- Sleep hygiene is the first step to fixing your sleep, which will impact your other symptoms.
- Mindful eating can substantially improve digestion.
- Energy conservation and pacing can be difficult but will help you retain the energy deposits you will make in the coming chapters.
- Mindset plays a big role in how successful we are at achieving our goals.
- There are many exercise options–if you aren't able to tolerate it now, come back to it.
- Make sure you begin practicing the foundations of healing before moving on!

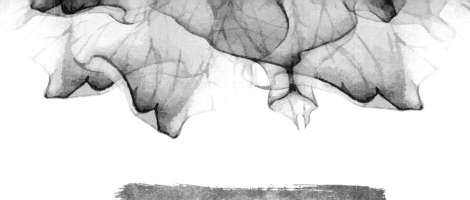

# CHAPTER 7

# SYMPTOM TRIGGERS

Now that you have begun your health journey with the foundations of healing, it's time to take a closer look at what may be triggering your symptoms. Over time, you will begin to identify specific events or situations that trigger your symptoms of pain, fatigue, and brain fog. These triggers tend to fall into one of three categories, which we will discuss in this chapter. It is impossible to avoid these triggers at all times, but awareness of them will be helpful in minimizing the effects they have on your health. It is ideal to work on minimizing these triggers for yourself as you undertake your health journey. Your health will improve much faster if you are not constantly triggered.

## DIET

Diet is a very important aspect of the treatment of fibromyalgia that rarely gets enough attention. Research has been performed on a variety of dietary alterations, including gluten-free, vegetarian, low-FODMAP, low calorie, and diets eliminating additives such as monosodium glutamate (MSG) and aspartame.[86] There is some evidence showing that highly inflammatory diets are associated with increased pain sensitivity in people with fibromyalgia.[87] Results of studies are mixed and far more research is needed. I suspect the inconclusive results are partially due to individual variation in which foods are inflammatory. Some of my patients with fibromyalgia feel fine eating gluten and dairy, whereas others notice significant changes in their symptoms with removal of these foods. Additionally, with repair to the digestive system, some people can eat foods they may not have tolerated previously.

Janet came to me with significant brain fog and moderate pain. She had quit her job as an accountant a few months earlier because she couldn't concentrate or perform the tasks she used to be able to. She felt as though fibro fog was robbing her of the career she had spent years in school for and absolutely loved. Janet was crushed when she felt she could no longer do her job well and resigned. She had been in a deep depression ever since. As we worked on identifying her symptom triggers, Janet eliminated gluten, wheat, dairy, nightshade vegetables, sugar, and food additives from her diet for three weeks (as described later in this chapter). When she reintroduced the foods she had eliminated, Janet noticed that gluten and sugar were major triggers for her brain fog. Janet hadn't realized how clear her mind had become since stopping these foods, but the fogginess and difficulty concentrating and processing information was very noticeable when she began consuming gluten and sugar again. She also realized that raw tomatoes and peppers increased her pain levels the day after she consumed them. Cooked tomatoes and peppers did not seem to have the same effect. Armed with this information, Janet could predict how she would feel after eating her food triggers and make an informed decision about whether the temporary pleasure was worth the consequences.

Determining your dietary triggers is a very individualized process. There are a few common culprits, including wheat- and gluten-containing foods, dairy products, nightshade vegetables (tomatoes, peppers, eggplant, and tobacco), high-sugar foods, food additives, and FODMAP-containing foods; however, you may have others. Based on what I've seen clinically, nightshade vegetables, food additives, and sugary foods are the biggest dietary contributors to increased pain levels in people with fibromyalgia. Gluten, wheat, and dairy tend to aggravate digestive symptoms or contribute to low energy levels and brain fog more than they affect pain. High-FODMAP foods can affect pain, energy, brain fog, and digestive symptoms; however, these foods often are not an issue once we've addressed digestive function. I've included instructions on how to determine your dietary symptom triggers below and a summary of the same in the *Additional Resources* section.

As general dietary advice to follow no matter what diet you are on or which stage of this process you are in, you'll want to apply the principles discussed in Chapter 6 regarding food choice. This is particularly important with protein. I recommend my patients consume a source of protein with every meal. If you are vegetarian or vegan, two servings of a plant-based protein will provide you with approximately the same amount of protein as one serving of animal-based protein. Protein helps stabilize blood sugars, gives your body the necessary building blocks to repair tissues, keeps you feeling fuller longer, and keeps energy levels higher. In the typical Western diet, protein often gets replaced with carbohydrates, which cause big changes in blood sugars. With frequent spikes and dips in blood sugar, you will experience cravings and energy crashes. It is also very important to minimize processed food. I know this can be incredibly difficult with fibromyalgia, since the energy and effort required to prepare food can be too much at times. Your food doesn't have to be complicated to be tasty and nutritious. Processed food will make your symptoms worse, and you will get stuck in a vicious cycle of feeling bad and eating processed food because it requires less effort, which in turn will make symptoms worse. If necessary, ask for help in getting your diet changes started.

## Elimination Diet

The process of doing an elimination diet involves following a restrictive diet for a short amount of time and then strategically reintroducing foods while monitoring symptoms to determine which foods cause you problems. It can be tedious, but it can give us answers we would not have found otherwise. As a general rule, you must follow an elimination diet for at least three weeks before reintroducing foods. The longest I will ever put a patient on a strict elimination diet is three months. Since the diet is restricted, there is a risk of nutrient deficiencies if it is followed long term. The elimination diet works best if it is paired with gut-healing strategies, which we will discuss in Chapter 10.

In my practice, I often give patients the choice of doing an elimination diet or taking the food sensitivity test described in the *Advanced Lab Testing* section of Chapter 4. In an ideal world with unlimited financial resources and motivation, I would recommend my patients do both, but we all know this is not an ideal world.

There are pros and cons to both the elimination diet and the food sensitivity test. As described in Chapter 4, the food sensitivity test measures an immune reaction (IgG antibodies) to food proteins. This means that your body has to elicit an immune response to a food for it to show up as abnormal on this test. It is possible to have reactions to food that do not involve an immune response, meaning these foods cause you symptoms, but you are not producing antibodies to the food itself. This is where the elimination diet comes in. When you do an elimination diet, we can determine which foods are causing symptoms, regardless of what your immune system is doing. We can pinpoint exact foods that are causing pain, brain fog, or fatigue that may not have shown up on the food sensitivity test. It also does not require much of a financial investment beyond what you spend on groceries. So why would I recommend you do both? We can't possibly eliminate every food from your diet. You do need to eat something. Plus, the food sensitivity test is quick and easy to do. You go to the lab, have your blood drawn, and a couple of weeks later we have a pretty lab report to review. The food sensitivity test is expensive, however, and may not be financially feasible for everyone. It also may not show the whole picture.

With an elimination diet, we can determine how you actually feel once we've removed suspected food triggers. We then challenge these foods and determine your symptomatic reaction to them. The main drawback of the elimination diet is that it is an involved process. It requires preparation, and you must pay attention to everything you eat while you're on it. Then, you must slowly reintroduce foods and track symptoms. The whole process can take up to three months or more. It's a time commitment and requires motivation to get through it. I've outlined the steps to follow for the elimination diet below. There is also a summary handout in the *Additional Resources* section.

**Note**: The elimination diet can be very triggering for people who are currently suffering from an eating disorder or those who have suffered from one in the past. If you have difficulty with disordered eating, I strongly recommend you skip this section or seek the advice of a health care provider prior to starting an elimination diet.

*Step 1: Determine Which Foods You Eat from the "Foods to Avoid" List.*

When looking at the elimination diet handout in the *Additional Resources* section, highlight the foods you eat that are listed in the *Foods to Avoid* column. These are the foods you are going to eliminate on your elimination diet. You can consume all of the foods listed in the *Foods to Eat* column, unless you have a known allergy or intolerance to anything listed here.

*Step 2: Make a Plan to Eliminate the Foods You Identified in Step 1.*

The elimination diet is easiest to follow if you plan your strategy in advance and ensure you have the foods on the *Foods to Eat* list available to you. Let's be honest, it is a tough diet, and anything you can do to make the process easier will be a huge help. I recommend to my patients that they make direct switches of foods where possible. For example, if you normally have cream in your coffee and yogurt for breakfast, switching to a plant-based milk for your coffee and a plant-based yogurt will be the least disruptive to your normal routine and will make this diet much easier. Examples of plant-based dairy alternatives allowed on the elimination diet are coconut milk and yogurt products. I know it doesn't quite taste the same, but many people discover they really enjoy plant-based dairy alternatives. I've included suggestions for easy switches you can make in the *Additional Resources* section.

As part of the preparation phase, I also recommend that you take an inventory of your symptoms and their severity. You can do this by listing your symptoms and rating them on a scale of 0 to 10, with 0 being no experience of the symptom and 10 being the worst severity of the symptom in question. Alternatively, you can use the WPI-SSS or FIQ questionnaires specific to fibromyalgia. I have included links to these questionnaires in the *Additional Resources* section. Improvement in symptoms can be gradual, and it may be difficult to remember how you felt at the beginning of the elimination diet, but having your symptoms recorded will give you a clear basis for comparison.

*Step 3: Eliminate the "Foods to Avoid."*

As discussed previously, the minimum amount of time you want to be on the elimination diet is three weeks. If your symptoms are severe and you are capable of following the elimination diet for longer, a timeframe of six weeks may be more useful. Since improvements are generally gradual, and it can be difficult to remember how you were feeling when you started the elimination diet, most people notice the biggest differences in symptoms in the reintroduction phase, when symptoms are retriggered by the offending food. If you are not noticing huge differences, be patient and stick with it.

Eliminating all of the foods you identified in Step 1 can be tricky if you already follow a more restricted diet, such as if you are vegetarian or vegan. It can also be tricky if the elimination diet is very different from how you normally eat. If this is the case for you, there are two ways you can do the elimination diet. The first way is to ease into the elimination diet by slowly cutting out food groups until you've cut out all of the *Foods to Avoid*, follow this for the desired amount of time (three weeks to three months), and then reintroduce the eliminated foods. The second way to do this is to eliminate the *Foods to Avoid* from one or two food groups for the desired amount of time (three weeks to three months), and then reintroduce these foods following the instructions in Step 5. You would then move on and eliminate the *Foods to Avoid* from the next one or two food groups for the prescribed amount of time and reintroduce these foods based on Step

5, and so on. In the second method, you are essentially doing several mini-elimination diets. The results will not be nearly as clear as they would be if you were to follow the full elimination diet, but if this is how it will work for you, you will likely gain some insight into your food triggers.

*Step 4: After the Elimination Phase, Prepare for the Reintroduction Phase.*

Once the time frame you decided on for the elimination phase is complete, rate your symptoms again in the same way you rated them at the beginning of the elimination phase in Step 2 (either on a scale of 0 to 10 or with the questionnaires). You can then compare these to how you felt at the beginning of the elimination phase but remember the biggest symptom differences are often noticed during the reintroduction phase. The reason for this is that when we are eating foods that generate inflammation in our bodies, it takes time for that inflammation level to come down and symptoms to decrease with it. When we challenge a food that causes inflammation in our digestive system, the effects (and resulting symptoms) are often quite obvious.

For the reintroduction phase, you will slowly reintroduce the foods you eliminated and track your symptoms as you do. I've included instructions on what information to include when tracking your symptoms in the *Additional Resources* section. I highly recommend that you write this information down! The reintroduction phase can be long, and it is difficult to remember which reactions you experienced from which foods once you get to the end. Having this information written down will also be helpful once you've completed gut healing, as you can then use it to determine if you are still experiencing the same symptoms from the food triggers you identified in the elimination diet.

Preparing for the reintroduction phase is similar to preparing to start the elimination phase. Ensure you go grocery shopping so that the foods you are going to reintroduce are available to you. Decide how you're going to track any symptoms that come up (see the *Additional Resources* section), and you are ready to move on to the next stage of the elimination diet!

*Step 5: Reintroduce the Foods You Were Avoiding and Track Any Symptoms That You Experience.*

To reintroduce the foods you were avoiding, you want to incorporate them slowly and in the purest form possible. For example, if you are reintroducing the dairy food group, start with a glass of milk. Once you've reintroduced milk (the purest form of dairy), you can move on to yogurt, then cheese, etc. For cheese, you will want to reintroduce each type of cheese that you regularly eat separately, since they are different foods, and some contain milk from different animals. This can get tricky with some food groups, but do your best with it. Avoid reintroducing two foods listed as *Foods to Avoid* at the same time. If you react to this combination, it will be impossible to tell which component you reacted to, and you will have to eliminate both again and then reintroduce them separately.

What do I mean by reintroducing foods slowly? This means that on day 1 of a food reintroduction, you will eat the reintroduced food three times. For the next three days (days 2 to 4), you will NOT consume the new food, and you will monitor symptoms. If you experience no symptoms from the reintroduced food, you can start consuming that food again as you please and reintroduce the next new food on day 5. If you did experience symptoms from that food, eliminate it until the end of the elimination diet, when you will challenge it a second time. If you experience symptoms from a food trigger, you must wait until the symptoms have resolved or settled back to your normal before reintroducing the next food.

Let's work through an example. Say you were reintroducing the vegetable group, specifically tomatoes. On day 1, you would consume tomatoes three times (ideally a portion of uncooked tomato). You would then avoid consuming anything containing tomatoes on days 2, 3, and 4. If you experienced no symptoms related to tomatoes, then on day 5 you can eat tomatoes as you normally would and reintroduce your next food. If you did experience symptoms from tomatoes, then you must avoid tomatoes for the rest of the reintroduction phase and wait until those symptoms resolve before reintroducing the next food. It can be helpful to write this out on a calendar as you go.

How do you choose which foods to reintroduce when? I usually recommend that people start with their favourite foods or the foods they miss most. It is ideal if you can reintroduce the *Foods to Avoid* from an entire food group before moving on to the next food group. For example, if you are really missing your yogurt for breakfast, then start with the dairy food group. Reintroduce milk first as described above, then yogurt, then cheese, etc. This makes the elimination diet more tolerable; however, many will disagree with my method. Many will recommend reintroducing the least inflammatory food first, then working towards the most inflammatory food (typically dairy, gluten, wheat, etc.). This would make your diet more variable faster, but most people's favourite foods fall in the category of more inflammatory foods. However you decide to reintroduce, it is helpful to write a list of the foods you are going to reintroduce in the order you plan to reintroduce them. You can change this order up slightly as you go, but it can be motivating to see your progress as you reintroduce foods you were avoiding.

*Step 6: Rechallenge the Foods That Caused Symptoms.*

Once you've gone through the reintroduction phase, you will very likely have a list of several foods that caused symptoms when you reintroduced them. You are going to challenge these foods a second time to determine whether they are still causing symptoms. Over the course of the elimination diet, you will have reduced the inflammation level in your gut and allowed some gut healing to occur. It is also possible that you were having an off day when you reintroduced that particular food (life happens), and it wasn't the food that was affecting your symptoms. Reintroduce the offending foods as per the instructions in Step 5 and determine if these foods are in fact a symptom trigger for you.

*Step 7: Continue to Avoid Foods That Caused Symptoms.*

If you've reintroduced a food twice and it still causes symptoms, then avoid the food. In some cases, once some gut healing has occurred, the food can be reintroduced into your diet with no problems. In other cases, you may have a tolerance level to a food, meaning you can consume small amounts with no problems, but larger amounts will cause symptoms. Finding this tolerance level can be tricky and requires trial and error. It is also possible to have symptoms from a raw food but not from the same food when it's cooked. You may decide that you don't enjoy this particular food that much and it's not worth the symptoms, or you may incorporate this food into your diet as a treat and consume it occasionally in smaller quantities. In less common instances, a food will always cause symptoms and cannot be reincorporated into your diet without causing distress. If this is the case for you, it is your decision whether you want to fully avoid the food and experience symptom relief or continue consuming it and live with the symptoms and inflammation it generates. When armed with this information, you can decide when consuming that food is worth it and be prepared for the consequences. If you go on to the gut-healing portion of digestive support discussed further in Chapter 10, then you will reintroduce the foods a third time after the gut-healing phase is complete.

*Step 8: Work on Gut Healing.*

We will go into detail on gut healing in Chapter 10, but I've included this step here so you are aware that some digestive support and gut lining repair may need to be done to optimize your digestion. There are a number of different supplements and herbs that we can use to stimulate proper digestion and heal the gut lining.

*Step 9: Rechallenge the Foods That Caused Symptoms After Completing Gut Healing.*

Utilizing the supplements and herbs discussed in Chapter 10 for gut healing generally takes about three to six months. They are not supplements or herbs that you need to take forever. After a three to six month course of gut healing and digestive support, most people experience much better digestion than they ever have in their entire lives. With proper diet, stress management, and avoidance of medications and substances that damage the gut, your digestive tract will remain healthy.

After completing gut healing, you will reintroduce for a third time the foods from the elimination diet that caused symptoms. Most often, you will not react to the food, since your gut lining is healed and the inflammation levels in your gut have decreased. If this is the case for you, you can reintroduce that food into your regular diet. If the food still causes symptoms it is best to avoid it, as the symptoms are a signal that this food is generating inflammation for you. If you decide to consume this food despite the symptoms, you now have the knowledge to make an informed decision about it.

## Low-FODMAP Diet

While I recommend that everyone go through the elimination diet at least once, the low-FODMAP diet has been researched specifically in people with fibromyalgia.[88] FODMAP stands for Fermentable Oligo-, Di-, and Mono-saccharides and Polyols. A mouthful, I know. Basically, FODMAPs are small, poorly digested carbohydrates that can lead to digestive symptoms, such as bloating, abdominal pain, diarrhea, constipation, and gas, in people who are sensitive to them.[89] Following the low-FODMAP diet has been shown to improve pain and digestive symptoms in people with fibromyalgia.[88] It is also used in the treatment of irritable bowel syndrome (IBS) and small intestinal bacterial overgrowth (SIBO).

I believe the reason that the low-FODMAP diet results in improvement in fibromyalgia symptoms is because of the link to gut bacteria imbalances, IBS, and SIBO. FODMAPs are carbohydrates that are perfect food for bacteria in the gut. An increase in food supply for the gut bacteria can lead to overgrowths and imbalances in the populations of these bacteria. In my experience, once the gut microflora population is corrected and SIBO is addressed (if present), people with fibromyalgia can happily eat FODMAP-containing food with no digestive issues or flares in fibromyalgia symptoms.

If you're not sure whether you have SIBO, but your digestive system is a mess, give the low-FODMAP diet a try and see how you feel. Improvements in symptoms can help you function better and make even bigger advances in your health. I've included the basics of the low-FODMAP diet below and a more detailed description in the *Additional Resources* section.

Garlic and onions are two of the biggest FODMAP offenders. Even if you are not highly sensitive to FODMAPs, you may still react to garlic and onions. If looking at the low-FODMAP diet handout in the *Additional Resources* section is giving you nightmares about the elimination diet, at least start with garlic and onions. Other foods containing FODMAPs are foods containing lactose, fructose, fructans (also known as inulin), galactans, and polyols. Examples of FODMAP-containing foods are some non-pitted fruits, honey, high fructose corn syrup, dairy products, wheat, beans, lentils, soy, fruits containing a pit (also known as stone fruits), sugar alcohols, and artificial sweeteners. This diet can be followed long term, used similarly to an elimination diet (with an elimination phase and a reintroduction phase), or used until the gut microflora have been rebalanced and the gut has been repaired.

## STRESS

We've discussed stress and its effects on fibromyalgia a few times throughout this book. Stress is one of the biggest symptom triggers you will be exposed to, and it won't always be avoidable. There are ways you can work to minimize stress and retrain your body to react to and cope with it in healthier ways. The ultimate goal is to retrain your body to engage in a situation-appropriate stress response and be able to shut the stress response off when it is not needed.

Our bodies respond to all types of stress in the same way, by generating inflammation, which in turn damages tissues and leads to poor functioning of our organ systems. Stressors can be physical, mental, or emotional. To our bodies, a stress is a stress is a stress. Negative emotions generate inflammation, just like eating an unhealthy diet.[90] This section will focus on emotional stress specifically, but keep this concept in mind as you are working on optimizing your diet and physical environment as well.

## Minimizing Unnecessary Stress

There are many things in life that we stress about unnecessarily. These things may be out of our control or may not actually involve us at all. They may involve family members, friends, or other people in the world. I applaud your kind and caring heart, but you need to focus on you and getting yourself to a healthier place. You may be able to do more about these stresses when you are feeling your best (if so, put them on your *One Day Visualization*!)

Take an account of your major stressors. Most people have three to five stressors that they would rate as major. Major stressors are stressors that disrupt your everyday life in some way. Maybe you think about them constantly, or they make you feel sad/angry/anxious/etc. Think about how much control you have over these stressors. Some you have more control over than others. You can also pass off some stressors or ask for help to minimize the amount of stress they cause. For example, if your house being messy is a major stressor for you, you can hire a housekeeper or assign housekeeping tasks to various members of your household to complete regularly. Finding ways to minimize your stressors will help significantly relieve symptoms.

Identify which stressors you have less or no control over. These are the stressors you need to let go of, at least for the time being. There may be a time when you have more control over these stressors, and you can then re-evaluate what you can do about them. For now, they are hindering your progress toward your main goal, which is to get to a place where you feel you are living well with fibromyalgia.

## Your Reaction to Stress

With fibromyalgia, your reaction to stress is abnormal. You feel it physically, and your body doesn't relax when it should. You live in this constant state of impending danger, leading to a state of depletion. With practice, you will learn to calm your body down and change your automatic reaction to stress.

When discussing the abnormal stress response in fibromyalgia and the ways this contributes to its symptoms, my patient Annabelle did not think this applied to her. She lived a relatively stress-free life compared to a lot of people she knew and as a result, didn't think she had an abnormal stress response. Annabelle had a stable and flexible job, no kids, a supportive partner, no major extended family stressors, and was financially comfortable. One weekend, Annabelle and her partner were visiting a couple they were friends with for dinner. The evening was going well, and they were all enjoying themselves, or so Annabelle thought. Partway through the dinner, the couple they were dining with became tense, and one partner raised his voice. Annabelle instantly felt on edge, despite the fact that his outburst was not directed at her. Her body tensed up and became more painful, she felt a headache coming on, and she started to feel panicky. It took Annabelle some time to recover. Her feeling of panic resolved within a few minutes once she removed herself from the situation and did some deep breathing in a calm space. She went to bed as soon as she got home, and the headache resolved the next day. Within a couple of days, the body pain had decreased back to the level it had been prior to the dinner. This made

Annabelle wonder if she truly did have an abnormal stress response, despite living a relatively stress-free life.

Pay attention to how you react when you are feeling stressed. Your reactions may be physical, mental, or emotional. Pausing throughout the day to take account of your stress level may be a helpful practice to draw your attention to your stress and work to minimize it. Telling your body out loud or in your head "I am safe" can work wonders in calming the stress response. Altering your reaction to stress will take practice, but being armed with the coping strategies we will discuss next will make the process much easier.

## Coping with Unavoidable Stress

Learning how to cope with stress in healthy ways is important for everyone. Unfortunately, much of our society has learned to cope with stress in unhealthy ways, including smoking, drinking, using drugs, eating too much or eating unhealthy food, or simply ignoring it. Learning healthy coping strategies will help decrease the stress-related symptoms you experience and prevent future flares of symptoms when stresses do inevitably arise.

### Counselling

I recommend professional counselling to many of my fibromyalgia patients if it is a feasible option for them. Going for counselling does not mean fibromyalgia is all in your head. There is most definitely a connection between your mental–emotional health and your physical symptoms, but that does not mean you are making your symptoms up.

Counselling can help you work through any past trauma you've experienced, develop healthy coping strategies, and assist you in working through any current emotional concerns. When we don't deal with our emotions properly, we internalize them, which leads to dysfunctions in our physiological processes. For example, if you have repressed anger from an instance (or series of instances) with your spouse that has not been processed and dealt with, this could contribute to your physical symptoms in the form of pain, headaches, and fatigue. It is important to be authentic to your emotions and allow yourself to feel them, but it's equally important to process those emotions and let them go. I've included two books on the connection between emotions/stress and physical well-being in the *Additional Resources* section if you are interested in learning more.

### Schedule Worry Time

A colleague of mine came up with the concept of scheduling worry time (Maggie Ackert, N.D., personal communication, 2018.) I love this idea! We have the tendency to allow our worries and stresses to invade every moment of every day when there is something bothering us. This gives these worries the power to rob us of every other aspect of our lives. When you are a person who tends to worry a lot about many different things, scheduling worry time can be a very helpful practice. Your worry time can be daily, weekly, or a few times a day, whatever works for you, as long as there are set boundaries around your worry time. For example, if you set your worry time at 10 minutes per day, you can use that 10 minutes to worry about whatever is on your mind, but once that 10 minutes is up, you put your worries away until your next worry time. If something comes up during the day that does not require your immediate attention, add it to the list for worry time. This is also a great time to worry about those stressors that are out of your control or big picture worries (such as global warming, world hunger, etc.).

## Meditation

We discussed meditation several times in Chapter 6, and I hope you've had a chance to practice some of those principles. Whether you're meditating before a meal, before bed, or periodically throughout the day, meditation is a skill that requires practice. It's highly unlikely that you will be a meditation pro in your first meditation practice.

Meditation looks different for different people. Some people enjoy deep breathing, while others enjoy listening to guided meditations (which come in a number of different forms), and still others find prayer or positive affirmations to be their ideal form of meditation. Yoga or movement paired with a meditation practice may be more your style. The point of meditation is to focus solely on relaxing, being in the moment, and taking a pause from the environment around you. The more often you can do this and induce a state of relaxation in your mind and body, the better you will be able to calm down your stress response and train your body to respond appropriately.

Meditation has been studied in people with fibromyalgia. In a study performed on mindfulness-based stress reduction in people with fibromyalgia, authors measured blood markers of the inflammatory response before and after an eight-week mindfulness program. These authors concluded that consistent mindfulness practices may help balance the inflammatory response in people with fibromyalgia.[94] Other research has measured the effects of mindfulness practices on fibromyalgia symptoms. Most studies show some benefit to symptoms, including improvements in pain, depression, anxiety, fatigue, and sleep quality; however, the studies are small and of mixed quality. Until more research is performed, it is difficult to draw definitive conclusions.[95–96]

Although we cannot definitively say based on research that mindfulness has a strong effect on the symptoms of fibromyalgia, meditation is easy to implement, can be practiced with no cost, and has minimal risk. Practicing mindfulness and meditation daily may be the key to achieving benefits, as research has been performed mainly on weekly practices. The more often you can train your body to enter a relaxed state, the easier it will be to do so when you are in a stressful situation. Continue working on finding a meditation that you can fully engage with and enjoy.

## ENVIRONMENT

The environment you find yourself in can either be a stress reliever or a stress inducer. Remember, your body processes all stressors the same way, and so it's not enough to reduce only your emotional stressors, it's also important to reduce your physical stressors. We've already covered diet in detail, and here we will examine what aspects of your physical and social environments may be triggering symptoms for you.

### Physical Environment

Your physical environment includes anything you are physically exposed to on a regular basis. There are a number of different areas we want to examine to ensure you are in the best physical environment possible to support your health journey. You will want to look for possible exposures in your home, work, and anywhere else you spend a significant amount of time. Exposure to toxic substances and chemicals means that your liver and kidneys have to work harder to detoxify those substances, and your detox pathways can become overwhelmed. Exposure to toxins can make symptoms of fibromyalgia worse or cause symptoms that you may be attributing to fibromyalgia.

## Mould

Visible mould anywhere is a problem. Mould can be present at home or at work. In people who are more sensitive, exposure to mould for even a short period of time can be problematic. If you see mould or suspect it is somewhere in your home or work environment, it needs to be investigated and dealt with appropriately. Mould is more likely to grow in moist environments, such as basements, on windowsills, or in areas that have ever been flooded. You can order petri dishes online to determine if you have mould in your environment. I have included the company I use in the *Additional Resources* section. If it is determined that you are being exposed to mould, it should be removed by a mould removal company. This can be very expensive. You should not use the same company for analysis of possible mould and for eradication of the mould. Continued exposure to mould can hinder any progress in your health, as your detoxification systems are already overloaded, and your body is not functioning well as a result.

## Plastics

Unfortunately, in our modern world almost everything is made of plastic. From a health standpoint, glass, metal, or fabric products are much better alternatives. The biggest issue with plastic is leaching of chemicals with major temperature changes, such as freezing or heating. This is most common with plastic water bottles if frozen or left outside in the sun, containers used to store or heat food, and shower curtains. Chemicals from plastics can significantly disrupt hormone balance and tax the detoxification systems in the liver and kidneys. The following guidelines will help you minimize your exposure to plastic:

- Where possible, switch food containers to glass or metal.
- Remove plastic shower curtains and replace with a fabric version.
- Use glass or metal water bottles and travel mugs.
- Use metal or glass straws, if applicable.

*Pesticides*

Many pesticides are endocrine-disrupting chemicals and are suspected to be linked to increased cancer rates.[91] An endocrine-disrupting chemical is one that disrupts hormonal balance within the body. Pesticide use is widespread and can be difficult to minimize without a big price tag. Organic foods do not have pesticides applied to them and typically show minimal pesticide residues on testing.[91] If it is possible for you, eating organic foods is the best option. If it is not financially feasible to eat all organic foods, consider the *Dirty Dozen, Clean 15* list published by the Environmental Working Group (EWG) every year.[92] The *Dirty Dozen* are the 12 foods that have the highest pesticide residues on testing. These are the foods you will get the greatest health benefit from by switching to the organic versions. The *Clean 15* are the 15 foods that have the lowest pesticide residues on testing. Buying the non-organic versions of these foods will not be as detrimental to your health and will save you from a substantial grocery bill. See the *Additional Resources* section for a link to the EWG website and to obtain your own copy of the *Dirty Dozen, Clean 15* list.[92]

*Cleaning and Beauty Products*

Similar to the food we eat, the products we use on our bodies and around our homes contain many harmful chemicals. Our skin is like a sponge and absorbs most of what we put onto it. Ensuring we are putting safe and more natural ingredients on our skin can significantly reduce our overall toxic burden. The products we use to clean our homes are products we're exposed to regularly and that we often unintentionally inhale. The EWG has a number of resources available to help you select healthier beauty and cleaning products, which I've included in the *Additional Resources* section.[94]

*Water*

What should be included in and excluded from drinking water is a controversial subject. On a basic level, drinking water should be clean and free from harmful bacteria. Tap water in many communities often contains harmful chemicals and metals.[97] More recently, media attention has been focused on the levels of lead in tap water. In older towns and cities, many of the water lines have not been replaced, and pipes carrying water to taps are still made of lead.[98] Governments have set limits on the allowable amounts of these chemicals; however, what is allowable and what is safe may not be the same.[99]

If you drink well water, you may be exposed to other minerals in high and possibly toxic amounts. The only way to know for sure is to have your water tested by a professional to determine what is in it. To avoid these potentially harmful elements in municipal tap or well water, using a water filter or purchasing spring water may be a better option. The EWG has developed a *Water Filter Guide* to help you choose a water filter.[100] A water filter doesn't necessarily need to be expensive to be effective. Do your research and find a solution that fits your budget. The links to the EWG's guides are in the *Additional Resources* section. For more information on what may be in your drinking water, you can contact your municipality or have your water tested by a third-party water analysis company.

## Social Environment

Your social environment can be just as toxic as your physical one. Have you ever had a friend or family member that consistently made you feel rotten? Or like you were always the one giving and never the one receiving? Relationships like that can be a huge emotional and energetic drain.

This issue is compounded by the fact that few people who do not have fibromyalgia understand what it is like to actually live with. This can leave you feeling unsupported, judged, and alone. But there is a difference between a lack of understanding and a lack of support. Friends and family members can be supportive, regardless of whether they completely understand your experience. There is a letter included in *The Complete Fibromyalgia Health, Diet Guide, and Cookbook* that has been helpful to many of my patients in explaining what it is like to live with fibromyalgia. This has helped them in determining who in their life is supportive and who isn't, as well as increasing understanding of their condition in their social circle.[101]

With respect to your social environment, it may be time to evaluate which relationships are good for you and which aren't. Taking a step back from an unhealthy relationship can give you time to evaluate what you need and want out of said relationship. You can determine whether it is likely that this relationship could be good for you or if it will always be an emotional and energetic drain. These emotional and energy-sucking relationships are called *toxic relationships*. They are relationships that take more effort than they are worth and give minimal return.

When you've cut toxic relationships from your life, you have more time and energy to focus on the good relationships in your life that both partners benefit from. Support from family and friends is very important in a condition like fibromyalgia. Support from others with fibromyalgia may be equally important. It's nice to know there are others you can relate to and ask questions when you're not sure about something related to your condition. There are a number of fibromyalgia support groups on Facebook and in-person. See the *Additional Resources* section for more information on finding a support group near you.

## KEY POINTS

- Symptom triggers can include foods, emotional stress, physical environment, and social environment.
- Doing an elimination diet can help you identify foods that trigger your symptoms.
- Common food triggers include wheat, gluten, FODMAP-containing foods, dairy products, nightshade vegetables, high-sugar foods, and food additives, such as aspartame and MSG.
- The low-FODMAP diet has been studied in fibromyalgia and was shown to reduce pain levels.
- Take an inventory of your stressors and work on minimizing your stress.
- It's equally important to learn to react to stress in a healthy way.
- Investigate your physical environment for possible symptom triggers, which could include exposure to mould, plastics, pesticides, cleaning and beauty products, and chemicals in drinking water.
- Minimize your exposure to toxic social environments and relationships when possible.

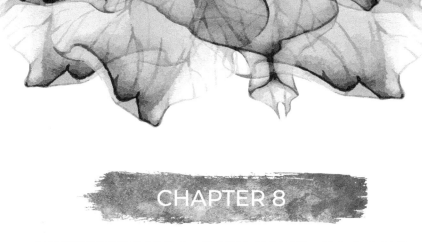

# CHAPTER 8

# NUTRITIONAL BUILDING BLOCKS

Understanding and removing aspects of your life that trigger your symptoms will help you make progress faster. Ensuring your body has basic nutritional components in appropriate amounts is another foundation we need to have in place before we work on more advanced nutritional strategies. If a nutritional deficiency has been identified on lab work, or your medications are depleting nutrients and they are not being replaced, this will be a huge barrier to your progress. We discussed common nutrient deficiencies that occur with fibromyalgia in Chapter 2.

Which nutrients you need will vary depending on your lab results, medications, and symptoms. It is ideal to work with a health care provider to determine which nutrients you should be supplementing. This is especially true for nutrients that can reach toxic levels by supplementation, such as iron and vitamin D. Dosing of iron and vitamin D should be based upon a lab value.

As for nutrient depletion caused by medication, I have included a resource in the *Additional Resources* section called Mytavin.[102] This database was developed by a medical doctor and is very user-friendly. To use this database, most often you need to know the pharmaceutical drug name of the medication you are on, not the brand or trade name. The brand or trade name of a drug can vary depending on what country you are in, but the pharmaceutical drug name should be consistent. For example, if you are taking Gravol (trade name), you would input dimenhydrinate as the drug name. If you are not sure what the drug name is, check the label of the product you are using or ask your pharmacist. Your pharmacist may also be able to check for nutrient depletion from medication.

If you are deficient in more than two common nutrients, you do not eat a balanced diet, or you feel overloaded with pills, it may be a good idea to take a multivitamin supplement rather than supplementing individual nutrients. Multivitamin supplements vary widely in terms of quality and dosing of ingredients. If you are going to spend money on a multivitamin, make sure it is good quality and contains nutrients in therapeutic doses. We will discuss multivitamins in more detail later in this chapter.

To determine whether a supplement is good quality, there are a few things you want to look for. First, has the supplement been tested by a third party? Third-party testing means that the supplement company has hired a company with no financial interest in selling the product to test the supplement for purity and accuracy of ingredients. Essentially, this third party is testing whether the supplement contains what is on the label in the dose listed. This helps to ensure that the supplement you are buying actually contains what it says it does. This information is often found on the company's website. You'll also want to choose a supplement that contains the active form of the ingredient you're looking for, if applicable. The most common example this applies to B vitamins, specifically vitamin B12 and folate. The methylcobalamin form of vitamin B12 and the 5-methyltetrahydrofolate form of folate are ready to use and don't require any additional conversion by the body. Lastly, you want to make sure that there are no *extras* in your supplement. Examples of extras can include gluten, wheat, soy, dairy, eggs, nuts, sugar, preservatives, artificial colour, or artificial flavouring. These ingredients are often listed in the *non-medicinal ingredients* section. Additionally, you can opt to choose products that are certified organic, non-GMO, vegan/vegetarian, and friendly to animals (if applicable, such as with fish oil products). If a supplement satisfies these criteria, there will be a certification on the label. A supplement doesn't necessarily have to be expensive, but make sure you're getting what you're paying for.

## POSSIBLE NUTRIENTS THAT MAY REQUIRE SUPPLEMENTATION IN FIBROMYALGIA

### B Vitamins

Most of the B vitamins play a vital role in energy metabolism. They act as very important cofactors for the enzymes involved in these processes. Symptoms of B vitamin deficiency can vary depending on which of the B vitamins are deficient, but could include fatigue, anemia, numbness, tingling, nerve pain, depression, skin rashes, rashes around the mouth, swollen tongue, poor memory, inability to concentrate, heart rate changes, muscle weakness, and irritability, among other symptoms.[103] Deficiency is not particularly common in North America, but it is possible. Following a vegetarian, vegan, or gluten-free diet or taking medications that deplete B vitamins may increase your risk of a deficiency.

Many of the B vitamins can be supplemented individually, and this may be the best option for you. If you suspect you are deficient in several B vitamins, or you are on medications that deplete B vitamins, a B-complex supplement may decrease the number of pills you need to take to replenish these nutrients. When choosing a B-complex supplement, ensure that the supplement contains all of the B vitamins (thiamine, riboflavin, niacin, pantothenic acid, biotin, folate, and vitamin B12).

Some B vitamins are available in multiple forms, and which one you choose may make a difference in how effective the supplement is for you. Folate comes in a synthetic form called folic acid. The folic acid form must be converted by the body to the active form prior to use. Folate also comes in a form that is ready for immediate use by the body, without additional conversion. When choosing a B-complex or a multivitamin, look for one that includes methyltetrahydrofolate (MTHF) on the label. MTHF is the active form of folate that your body can use without conversion. Some individuals have a genetic defect in the pathway converting folic acid to MTHF and as a result, cannot convert the synthetic form of folate to the active form. The only way to know for sure whether this affects you is to have genetic testing.

Vitamin B12 also comes in a number of different forms. The least expensive form of vitamin B12 is cyanocobalamin, and this form is common in supplements. Cyanocobalamin is a synthetic form of vitamin B12, and the body must convert it to an active form before it can be used. When choosing a B vitamin supplement, choose a supplement containing vitamin B12 in the forms of methylcobalamin, hydroxycobalamin, or adenosylcobalamin. All three of these forms of vitamin B12 are present naturally in the body and can be used without conversion.

Each of the B vitamins is required in different amounts, so choosing a B-complex with 100mg or 50mg of each B vitamin may not be the best option. Dosing of individual B vitamins can also vary depending on what you are trying to accomplish. Consult with your health care provider to determine the best doses for you. Possible adverse effects of supplementation with B vitamins include stomach upset, diarrhea, facial flushing, rash, heartburn, nausea, vomiting, headache, or dizziness.[61,104–110] Many people experience bright yellow urine with B vitamin supplementation, and this is normal. To minimize adverse effects and maximize absorption, take B vitamins with food.

## Magnesium

Magnesium is a nutrient that is commonly deficient in people living in North America.[111] This is in part due to a diet lacking in magnesium-rich food, such as nuts and leafy vegetables.[111] The typical North American diet contains many grain products, which do not provide much magnesium. Compounding this problem are deficiencies in the soil in which we grow our food. Typically, plants absorb nutrients such as magnesium from the soil, but most of the soil we use is depleted of magnesium, resulting in lower magnesium content in the food we eat.

Magnesium comes in a variety of forms. The less expensive forms that are often contained in lower quality magnesium supplements are magnesium oxide and magnesium chloride. These forms are more likely to cause digestive upset and should be avoided where possible.[111] The forms of magnesium I use most often in my practice are magnesium bisglycinate, magnesium malate, and magnesium citrate. Magnesium bisglycinate can have a calming effect due to the effects of glycine in the bisglycinate portion and is useful with muscle pain and cramping.[112–113] This form of magnesium has not been specifically studied in fibromyalgia, but I find it very helpful for pain reduction, as well as for improving sleep and mood. Magnesium malate has been studied specifically in fibromyalgia. This form of magnesium was shown to decrease pain in people with fibromyalgia in a small study.[114] Both magnesium and malic acid are involved in ATP-generating pathways, which may be why they show benefit in fibromyalgia. Doses that appeared to be most effective were 400mg daily of magnesium and 1600mg daily of malic acid continued for at least two months.[114] Magnesium citrate tends to have more effects on the bowels and is useful in addressing constipation. Magnesium will be discussed further in Chapter 9.

## Iron

As mentioned previously, it is possible to be iron deficient without the presence of an anemia. Within the body, iron makes up the portion of red blood cells responsible for carrying oxygen to the cells. Iron also acts as a cofactor for many enzymes. Iron deficiency can result in a variety of symptoms including anemia, restless leg syndrome, depression, fatigue, heart palpitations, pale skin, impaired cognitive performance, decreased resistance to infection, and impaired ability to maintain body temperature.[103,115] It is possible to overload on iron and this can be toxic, so supplementation with iron should be monitored with regular blood work. Dosing of an iron supplement should always be based on lab results.

Where possible, it is preferable to get iron from food rather than a supplement. There are two forms of iron in food, heme and non-heme. Heme iron is the form of iron that is present in meat products, and this form is more bioavailable to the body. Non-heme iron is the form present in plant-based foods and is less bioavailable to the body. For this reason, the people at highest risk of iron deficiency include people following a vegetarian or vegan diet, as well as menstruating and pregnant women. Low stomach acid can also contribute to development of an iron deficiency.

Consuming meat products is not the only way to boost iron levels with food. Cooking food, specifically acidic food, in cast-iron pans can help increase the iron content of the food.[116] Consuming iron-rich food or supplements with a source of vitamin C can also help increase iron absorption.[115] When trying to increase iron levels, avoid taking iron supplements or eating iron-rich food alongside coffee, tea, or supplements containing zinc or magnesium.[115] Possible adverse effects of iron supplementation include stomach upset, abdominal pain, constipation, diarrhea, nausea, and vomiting.[117] The most common adverse effect is constipation. This can be minimized by slowly increasing the iron supplement dose to the target dose over several weeks and by addressing stomach acid levels. See the *Additional Resources* section for details on how to increase doses.

## Vitamin D

Vitamin D can be obtained from sunlight; however, this is only possible when the UV index is three or higher, and a sufficient amount of unprotected skin is exposed for an appropriate amount of time.[118] Since Canada and a portion of the United States do not get enough sunlight at appropriate strength for a good portion of the year, many people are vitamin D deficient. Vitamin D is also present in some foods, but amounts are not high enough to prevent a deficiency. Your vitamin D status can be determined using a blood test.

Vitamin D plays an important role in cognition, immune health, bone health, and mood, and is suspected to play a role in sleep quality.[118]

Symptoms of vitamin D deficiency can include bone loss and fractures, bone pain, depression, muscle pain, muscle cramping or weakness, and fatigue.[119] Vitamin D has been researched as a possible treatment option in people with fibromyalgia. Vitamin D deficiency in fibromyalgia appears to be associated with ratings of pain and quality of life, as well as levels of anxiety and depression.[120] People with fibromyalgia who were deficient in vitamin D experienced more pain, headache, depression, and sleep dysfunction.[120] When the vitamin D deficiency was corrected, symptoms of fibromyalgia improved. However, symptoms of fibromyalgia did not improve with vitamin D supplementation if there was no deficiency prior to initiating supplementation.[121] There is little consensus on appropriate dosing of vitamin D to correct a deficiency; however, dosing should be based on an lab value of 25-hydroxyvitamin D.

Vitamin D3 is the best form of vitamin D to supplement with, as this is the form most effectively used by the body. When supplementing with vitamin D, it is ideal to take it daily with a meal containing some fat. I recommend my patients use a vitamin D3 supplement that is in either a gel capsule or oil form. Tablet forms are not ideal for vitamin D supplementation. Dosing of a vitamin D supplement should always be based on a lab result. Vitamin D can reach toxic levels, and vitamin D toxicity can be dangerous. Always seek the advice of a health care provider prior to starting a vitamin D supplement or consuming large doses.

## Multivitamins

Multivitamins are not useful for everyone. I only use multivitamins in the treatment of specific diseases, when a very restrictive diet is followed, or when there are more than two nutrient deficiencies we are aiming to correct. In the case of correcting several nutrient deficiencies, the use of a multivitamin supplement should be considered when it decreases the number of pills you must take. Otherwise, it is preferable that you be more targeted in your nutrition support.

When choosing a multivitamin, it is ideal to choose one that contains both vitamins and minerals but no other extra ingredients. Many multivitamin supplements contain herbs, which are often present in doses too small to have any effect and only increase the possibility of medication interactions. As described above, you are looking for a multivitamin that undergoes third-party testing, contains ingredients in the active forms, and contains no extra ingredients that you could react to.

## KEY POINTS

- It is important to make sure the body has the basic building blocks it needs before adding more sophisticated supplemental support.
- Determining whether you are deficient in any of the nutritional building blocks may require lab testing.
- Proper dosing of some nutritional building blocks may also require a lab value.
- Supplement with individual nutrients unless you have a specific reason for using a multivitamin.
- If you're going to spend money on supplements, choose good-quality ones.

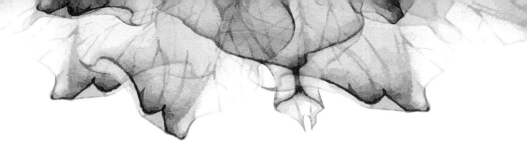

SECTION 3

# Advanced Treatment of Fibromyalgia

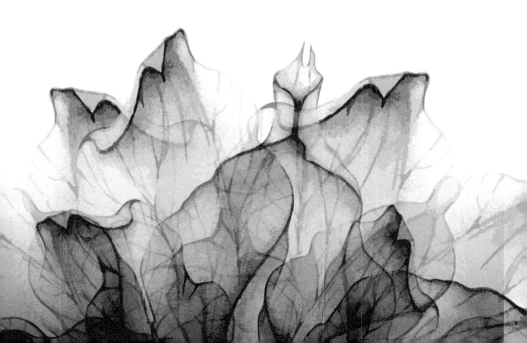

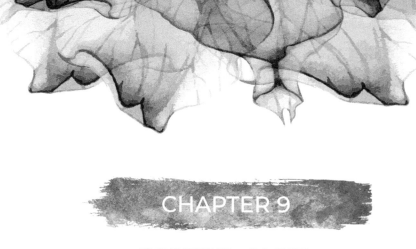

# CHAPTER 9

# RESTFUL SLEEP

With the foundations of healing in place, it's time to discuss sleep. Addressing sleep problems will be some of the most important work you do for your fibromyalgia symptoms. As discussed in Chapter 6, sleep in fibromyalgia is lighter and more fragmented than sleep in people without fibromyalgia.[8,25,79] This means you wake frequently during the night and wake in the morning feeling unrefreshed. You are not getting the deep, restorative sleep that allows your brain to fully rest and your body the ability to heal itself. The cause of brain wave abnormalities during sleep in fibromyalgia is not known, but I suspect the abnormal stress response is at the heart of the issue. Brain inflammation, as discussed in the study referenced in Chapter 2, could also play a role.[8,31]

Practicing the lifestyle habits outlined in Chapter 6 is the first step toward fixing this problem. Sleep hygiene is very important in allowing the body to prepare for sleep and in separating the day's activities from sleep time. Continuing to practice meditation, as part of your bedtime routine and/or at other times throughout the day, is also immensely helpful in calming the body's stress response and allowing for deep, restorative sleep.

## Natural Support for Restful Sleep

Supplemental melatonin is the most well-known option for natural sleep support. I find that melatonin alone is often not enough to support sleep in people with sleep difficulties and in fibromyalgia, but in some cases it is useful. There are a handful of natural sleep support options I use regularly, depending on what is disrupting sleep.

*Melatonin*

Melatonin is produced naturally by the brain in response to darkness and is suppressed in response to light. Melatonin has a variety of functions in the body but is most well-known for its role in sleep. As an added bonus, melatonin has been shown to reduce pain levels in a number of painful conditions.[122] It is produced from the amino acid tryptophan, which is made into serotonin and then melatonin. As discussed in Chapter 2, there appear to be abnormalities in the tryptophan–serotonin pathway, which could point to issues with melatonin production.[8,31] Melatonin can also be depleted by a number of medications, which can further disrupt sleep. As a supplement, melatonin can be dosed from 0.5mg to 20mg daily depending on what condition is being treated, with doses in the 3–5mg range most commonly used.[122]

Supplemental melatonin comes in two forms, immediate release and sustained release. Most melatonin supplements are immediate release, unless they are specifically labelled sustained release or prolonged release. Immediate-release melatonin will help you fall asleep faster when you go to bed. Sustained-release melatonin can be used to prevent you from waking during the night but is less helpful at decreasing the amount of time it takes you to fall asleep.

To be effective as a sleep agent, melatonin must be taken about 30–60 minutes before bedtime. A number of adverse effects are possible with melatonin use, including headache, dizziness, nausea, and a feeling of drowsiness on waking.[122] With high doses of melatonin or in people who are particularly sensitive, nightmares and very vivid dreams are a possible adverse effect. Since melatonin can be highly effective at inducing drowsiness, it is recommended that you avoid driving or operating heavy machinery for five hours after taking it. Melatonin also interacts with a number of different medications, so be sure to check with your health care provider prior to use if you are taking any medication.

I rarely use melatonin alone as sleep support. I do not find it to be effective enough on its own to correct sleep dysfunction, resulting in the use of higher and higher doses and more adverse effects. I also find that the effects of melatonin vary from person to person. Clinically, I've seen some people experience an opposite reaction to melatonin. Instead of melatonin making them drowsy, it makes them feel wired or have more difficulty sleeping than they did previously. Generally, I like to use melatonin in combination with other sleep-supportive agents.

In treating fibromyalgia, I often start with a supplement containing melatonin along with L-theanine and 5-HTP, both of which we'll discuss. The combination I use comes as one chewable tablet containing 1.5mg of melatonin with 100mg of L-theanine and 15mg of 5-HTP (5-hydroxytryptophan). The dose of this formulation is 1–2 tablets about 30 minutes before bed. I always recommend starting with a ½ tablet to see how you tolerate it. A number of different brands carry this same formulation, and it should not be too difficult for you to find. This combination is most effective if stress, anxiety, and worry are preventing you from falling asleep or if you wake during the night feeling anxious or worried.

On a cautionary note, 5-HTP should **not** be used with certain antidepressant medications, specifically ones that alter serotonin levels in the brain. This can lead to the development of a condition called serotonin syndrome, which can be fatal. Please always check with your health care provider if you are unsure whether a supplement interacts with your medication.

An exception to the guideline of not using melatonin alone is if you wake frequently in the night but have no difficulty falling asleep when you go to bed. This sleep pattern is less common than difficulty falling asleep at bedtime or experiencing both difficulties falling asleep and waking frequently during the night. If you have already tried adding in a bedtime snack containing protein and natural sugars, and you are still waking during the night, adding sustained-release melatonin can be incredibly effective at keeping you asleep throughout the night.

*Theanine and 5-HTP*

Theanine is an amino acid that is present in green tea. As a supplement, it is used to relieve worry and anxiety, as well as improve cognitive performance. It can be used on its own or in combination with other supplements. Doses typically range from 100–200mg per day.[123] Adverse effects from taking theanine are rare but can include headache or sleepiness.[123]

As described above, I use theanine in combination with other sleep supports when addressing sleep dysfunction. Theanine on its own also works wonderfully during the daytime for anxiety, as it does not make most people feel sleepy. It works quickly and can be used as needed for stressful events or for day-to-day anxiety treatment. Theanine is very safe and does not interact with many drugs.[123]

5-HTP (hydroxytryptophan) is produced within the body from tryptophan. 5-HTP is used to make serotonin and melatonin, making it a useful treatment option for both sleep and mood disorders. 5-HTP is rarely used as a sleep-supportive supplement on its own. However, it is commonly used to address depression and anxiety alone or in combination with other natural treatments.[124] Doses of 5-HTP range from 100–900mg daily, although I recommend 15–30mg nightly in combination with theanine and melatonin.[124]

When I first met Camila, she was sleeping about two hours per night in divided amounts. She felt awful and was sick of trying to fight through the exhaustion. When she couldn't sleep, her mind was racing with thoughts of work, the kids, and how she was going to get through the next day. Even when she'd had a bad night's sleep the night before, she still couldn't sleep. I recommended this blend of melatonin, L-theanine, and 5-HTP at a starting dose of a ½ tablet 30 minutes before bed to help her fall asleep and get longer periods of sleep. Camila came back two weeks later and said she had to stop taking the tablets, because they were knocking her out. She was sleeping deeply for six hours straight, and that scared her. We decreased Camila's dose to a ¼ tablet 30 minutes before bed to see how she would do. Camila tolerated the ¼ tablet dose much better. She found she could sleep for five to six hours at a time and didn't wake up feeling like a zombie.

Possible adverse effects from the use of 5-HTP are typically digestive in nature, including nausea, vomiting, abdominal pain, diarrhea, and loss of appetite.[124] Adverse digestive effects are typically relieved by taking a supplement with food; however, more sensitive people may experience adverse effects even when a supplement is taken with food. As mentioned above, 5-HTP can interact dangerously with some medications. If you are on medication, please ensure 5-HTP is safe for you before consuming.

## Magnesium

Magnesium is one of the supplements I use the most in my practice. It plays a role in over 300 reactions in the body and helps regulate a large number of bodily functions.[112] Magnesium is very effective in treating sleep dysfunction, anxiety, digestive conditions, and pain conditions. Deficiency in magnesium is widespread and cannot be measured through blood testing. Magnesium is one of my top supplements for fibromyalgia, as long as it is tolerated.

There are a number of different forms of magnesium that are used for different reasons. While magnesium itself helps relieve pain, calm emotions, and relax the body, we can get added benefit from different compounds magnesium may be bound to in a supplemental form. The form I most commonly see patients using when they come into my office is magnesium citrate. Magnesium citrate is great for treating constipation and irregular bowel habits. Since magnesium citrate tends to stimulate bowel movements, it is more likely to cause diarrhea than other forms of magnesium.

There are two forms of magnesium I find most effective in fibromyalgia: magnesium malate and magnesium bisglycinate. Magnesium malate has been researched in fibromyalgia and may help reduce pain.[114]

Malate (also known as malic acid) and magnesium are found in the mitochondria, and both play a role in the formation of energy molecules within our cells.[114]

Magnesium bisglycinate is useful in treating muscle tension, muscle cramping, sleep disorders, and anxiety. In the magnesium bisglycinate form, magnesium is attached to glycine.[113] Glycine is an amino acid that has a calming effect on the nervous system and decreases core body temperature slightly, which helps make us sleepy.[113]

Dosing of oral magnesium typically ranges from 200–400mg of elemental magnesium daily.[125] Possible adverse effects tend to be digestive in nature, including stomach upset, diarrhea, nausea, and vomiting.[125] Magnesium is best absorbed if taken with food; however, many people do well taking magnesium before bed without food. If you have low blood pressure, taking magnesium may lower it further, resulting in dizziness or fainting.[125]

Adding a magnesium supplement was life changing for Rhonda. Rhonda experienced severe muscle soreness and frequent headaches that turned into migraines if she didn't address them quickly enough. We added two forms of magnesium to Rhonda's plan. Rhonda started taking a magnesium malate supplement in the morning and a magnesium bisglycinate supplement shortly before bedtime. She had her first headache-free day in years. Rhonda's headaches decreased by 60% within six weeks of starting magnesium. Muscle pain was no longer keeping Rhonda awake at night, either. She could find a comfortable position in bed, sleep through the night, and was less sore on waking.

In practice, I use a supplement that combines the three forms of magnesium discussed here: magnesium citrate, magnesium bisglycinate, and magnesium malate. I find this supplement useful in fibromyalgia, since it addresses pain, fatigue, and sleep dysfunction, and often helps with the bowel symptoms that accompany fibromyalgia. This supplement is also available in liquid form, allowing for a wide variety of doses and the ability to find a dose that is well tolerated by the patient. Magnesium has interactions with a number of drugs, some of which can be serious. Be sure to check with your health care provider prior to starting this supplement.

*Passionflower*

Passionflower is an herb that acts to calm the body and can make some users sleepy.[126] Passionflower has not been specifically studied in fibromyalgia. I use passionflower often because it tends to be well tolerated, and it does not interact with many medications.[126] Most users find it calming, without being too sedating. It helps with sleep but doesn't make you feel like a zombie. This herb is particularly useful when worry and anxiety are preventing you from falling asleep, you are waking during the night from worry, or if drug interactions are a concern with other sleep supports. It works well in people who experience panic attacks and can used on an as-needed basis or as a daily support.

Passionflower is available in a standardized pill form, as a tincture, or as a tea. I use the tincture form most often, as it allows for more flexibility in dosing, and I find it to be more clinically effective. If you are particularly sensitive to new supplements, you may want to try a tea form first. The capsule form of passionflower is typically dosed from 40–200mg daily, on an empty stomach if tolerated.[126] The dosing of the tincture form depends on the strength of the product, which should be taken as directed on the label.

Possible adverse effects of passionflower include dizziness, sedation, and confusion.[126] When trying this supplement for the first time, I recommend taking it shortly before bedtime to determine how sleepy it makes you feel. Anything you take orally carries the risk of digestive upset, particularly if you are sensitive to supplements. If you experience digestive upset with passionflower, try taking it with food to see if that negates the adverse effects.

### Valerian

Valerian is a strong sleep-inducing herb. I add valerian only when we've tried the other combinations listed above, and we still cannot regulate sleep. Valerian can be used to decrease the amount of time it takes to fall asleep and to help prevent nighttime wakening. I find valerian to have strong sedative properties, and as such it is not effective for addressing anxiety during the daytime. This herb works well alone or in combination with other sleep supports, particularly passionflower.

Valerian comes in capsule form, tincture form, and tea form. A tincture is an alcohol extract of herbs. Valerian has a very distinct smell, similar to dirty gym socks. This can make it difficult to take as a tea or tincture. Clinically, I find that valerian works well in all forms as long as it is tolerable to the individual. Doses of valerian in the range of 400–900mg within two hours of bedtime appear to be the most effective for falling asleep faster and improving sleep quality.[127] Possible adverse effects of valerian use include headache, stomach upset, mental dullness, dry mouth, vivid dreams, and morning drowsiness.[127] Similar to melatonin, some people have an opposite reaction to valerian than expected. Rather than valerian inducing a sleepy and calm feeling, the users feel wired and cannot sleep. Valerian interacts with a number of medications, and caution should be exercised if starting this supplement alongside medication.[127]

## KEY POINTS

- Combinations of sleep agents often have better effects on sleep than single ingredients.
- Sustained-release melatonin can help prevent waking through the night but is less effective for falling asleep more quickly.
- Melatonin in combination with theanine and 5-HTP works well for sleep disrupted by anxiety, worry, or difficulty turning your brain off.
- Passionflower can also be used when anxiety or worry are disrupting sleep or as daytime anxiety support.
- Valerian is a strong sedative and can help with falling asleep and staying asleep.

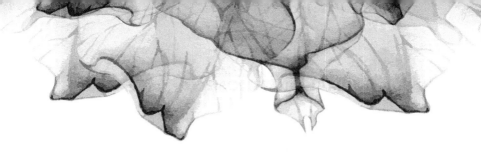

# CHAPTER 10

# OPTIMIZING DIGESTION

Next to proper sleep, optimizing digestive function will have the greatest impact on your symptoms. Proper functioning of the gut is vital to health. If we can't digest food and absorb nutrients, we can't make energy, repair tissues, recover from injuries or illness, or grow and get stronger. We can't function optimally if our digestive system isn't functioning optimally. Often, our digestive systems have been functioning poorly for so long that we accept our symptoms as normal. As you know, there are many digestive symptoms and conditions that correlate with having fibromyalgia. Some of those conditions have specific treatment plans that are not covered here (SIBO, for example), but what we'll discuss here will apply to many of you. I want digestive discomfort to be a distant memory for you.

# WHAT IS NORMAL DIGESTION?

When asked, many people cannot articulate what is normal in terms of digestion. This is an important place to start. How do you know if what you're experiencing is abnormal if you don't even know what normal is? While there is some variation in normal, there are some basics we want to aim for with digestion.

Digestion should be a comfortable process. So comfortable, in fact, that you are largely unaware that it's occurring. You should not have any abdominal pain, discomfort, or excessively noisy digestion. You should not experience bloating or gas pain. Some gas and burping are normal but should not be excessive or uncomfortable. Passing gas about 14 to 23 times per day is considered normal.[128] Burping is more likely to occur with consumption of carbonated beverages, and this is normal. There should be no instances of heartburn or food regurgitation. Nausea and vomiting should not occur on a regular basis. You should have one to three bowel movements per day. Bowel movements should be comfortable, without straining or pain. You should feel the urge to have a bowel movement but should not have to run to the toilet to avoid having an accident. There should be no blood, mucus, or undigested food (other than corn) in your stool. Stools should be formed and not watery or hard.

How many of those criteria did you check off as normal? We want to aim to have them all in place or as close to the normal range as possible. There are a number of reasons why your digestion could be far from normal. If your symptoms are severe, it's important to be evaluated by a health care professional to ensure you don't have a more serious condition that requires more involved treatment and monitoring. If you've been given the all clear, or your symptoms are annoying but not severe, the tips listed in the rest of the chapter may be for you.

## DISCOVERING YOUR GUT PROBLEM

The symptoms you experience and when you experience them can point us in a specific direction as to where your digestive system is not functioning well. For example, symptoms that occur while eating signal a problem in the upper digestive tract, including issues in the mouth, esophagus, or stomach. Symptoms that occur about 30 minutes to one hour after eating are typically related to the small intestine. If symptoms occur more than one hour after eating, this signals an issue in the large intestine or colon.

Specific symptoms themselves also tend to give us clues about where we can work to optimize digestion. The symptoms of heartburn and food regurgitation signal imbalances in stomach acid levels that need to be corrected for digestion to begin on the right note. Bloating and gas occur when undigested food passes through the digestive tract and reaches an area where the gut bacteria have a feeding frenzy. When gut bacteria eat the undigested food, they produce gas. Depending on where the gas is produced, it can become trapped and cause bloating, or it can be released and cause flatulence or burping. Digestive symptoms can also be caused by dysfunction in multiple areas of the digestive tract. Luckily, there are a few common patterns that are easy to correct.

## WHAT IS LEAKY GUT?

*Leaky gut* has been all the rage in the media in the past few years. While leaky gut is not an officially accepted diagnosis in the medical community, it is a phenomenon that has been observed by functional and alternative medicine practitioners. Leaky gut means exactly what the name implies: your gut is leaking and allowing things it shouldn't to pass from the digestive tract into the blood. This is also known as intestinal hyperpermeability.

Over time, different factors can cause inflammation in the gut. We've discussed most of these factors already. As a refresher, they could include poor food choices, consumption of foods you are sensitive to, medication, stress, or alcohol consumption. Normally, the gut lining is tight, and the cells are joined close together. When the gut is exposed to these factors and inflammation develops, gaps form between the cells. Instead of these cells creating a barrier to keep the contents of the digestive tract in, the lining now allows various substances to pass from the digestive tract into the bloodstream. Some of these substances are large or would not normally have made it through the lining of the digestive tract, which generates even more inflammation. To repair the gut lining, we need to remove the triggers causing inflammation. We discussed food sensitivities and eliminating food symptom triggers with the elimination diet in Chapters 4 and 7. This is the first step to repairing leaky gut. For strategies to heal the gut lining, see the *L-glutamine* and *Demulcent Herbs* sections later in this chapter.

## HYPOCHLORHYDRIA

One of the most common digestive dysfunctions I see in my practice is hypochlorhydria, also known as low stomach acid. Common symptoms of hypochlorhydria include heartburn, indigestion, abdominal pain, feeling of excessive fullness, bloating, and food or acid regurgitation.[59] Without appropriate levels of stomach acid, it is almost impossible to digest food properly. This leads to a host of other issues with digestion including low levels of digestive enzymes, gut bacteria imbalances, food intolerances, and increased risk of infection.[59] In my practice, I perform a simple test to determine whether stomach acid is low, so we can determine the appropriate treatment. This test is called the *Apple Cider Vinegar Challenge.*

## Apple Cider Vinegar (ACV) Challenge

The Apple Cider Vinegar Challenge is the test I use to determine whether stomach acid is low. High stomach acid, also known as hyperchlorhydria, can also cause heartburn and abdominal pain. Since treatment options for this are very different from those for low stomach acid, it is important to determine which we are dealing with. Conventionally, heartburn is always treated by lowering stomach acid. The treatment of choice in conventional medicine is a drug called a proton-pump inhibitor (PPI) or an antacid. Clinically, I see that heartburn and other digestive symptoms are much more commonly caused by low stomach acid, which requires that we raise stomach acid to correct the problem.

When I describe low stomach acid as being a cause of heartburn and other digestive concerns, many people are confused. Doesn't it make logical sense that high stomach acid would mean acid is escaping the stomach and causing a burning sensation in the esophagus? The answer is yes and no. In the rare case that stomach acid is high, it can cause many problems. When stomach acid is low, there is not enough acid produced to digest food properly. Additionally, without appropriate stomach acid levels there are no messages to close off the stomach from the esophagus. This is the job of the lower esophageal sphincter, which is a small circular muscle wrapped around the esophagus where it meets the stomach. When stomach acid is at an appropriate level, this circular muscle tightens and closes the opening of the stomach to prevent acid from leaking into the esophagus. When stomach acid is low, this circular muscle doesn't get the signal to tighten, allowing the passage of acid from the stomach into the esophagus and resulting in unpleasant symptoms, including heartburn.

To determine whether hyper- or hypochlorhydria is contributing to your digestive symptoms, the test is simple. Mix one tablespoon of apple cider vinegar into a small amount of water to create a shot. Take this mixture immediately before your biggest meal. If you experience **no** heartburn, burning in the chest, or abdominal pain, take this mixture immediately before every meal for two to three days. If you continue to tolerate the apple cider vinegar mixture well, you have low stomach acid. If you experience heartburn, burning in the chest, or abdominal pain, discontinue immediately, as this indicates you have normal or high stomach acid. If you determine that your stomach acid is low, discontinue the ACV after 3–4 days, and see the *Bitter Herbs* section of this chapter for how to repair your digestion.

## DIGESTIVE ENZYME DEFICIENCY

Digestive enzyme deficiency is rarely detected on standardized lab testing and is a symptom-based alternative medicine diagnosis. Deficiency in digestive enzymes typically goes hand in hand with low stomach acid. Symptoms of a digestive enzyme deficiency could include bloating, abdominal discomfort, gas, diarrhea or constipation, nausea, and fatigue. When digestive enzymes are not produced and released in sufficient amounts, your food is not digested properly. This can lead to undigested food passing through the digestive tract. As discussed previously, gut bacteria feed on this undigested food, leading to symptoms and potentially gut bacteria imbalances. With a digestive enzyme deficiency, it is possible that fat, protein, and carbohydrate digestion are all affected or that just one or two of the macronutrients aren't being digested properly. Most people can pinpoint which foods they have more trouble digesting, and this is likely because those are the enzymes that are affected.

## A Note on Digestive Enzymes

You may think that if you have a digestive enzyme deficiency, then you need to supplement with digestive enzymes. I rarely use digestive enzymes in my practice, except in very specific cases. Supplementing with digestive enzymes is a Band-Aid solution that does not fix the underlying problem. When you supplement with digestive enzymes, you are replacing what your body should be doing naturally, allowing your body to continue in this dysfunctional pattern. It is unlikely that you will be able to come off digestive enzymes, because the underlying issue will still be present.

## GUT BACTERIA IMBALANCES

It is possible to have imbalances in your gut bacteria and not have SIBO. Many people have imbalances in their gut bacteria, leading to generation of inflammation, digestive symptoms, and pain. It's a good idea to be investigated for SIBO if possible, as there is a strong link between SIBO and fibromyalgia.[74] If you don't have SIBO, adding a probiotic to your digestive treatment plan may be a great option. See the *Probiotics* section of this chapter for more guidance.

## HOW TO OPTIMIZE YOUR DIGESTION

While optimizing digestion is important, there is no combination of supplements that can fix a poor diet. It is important that you do the dietary work outlined in Chapter 7 before using the digestive system repair strategies outlined here.

## Bitter Herbs

If you have taken the ACV challenge and determined that your stomach acid is low, or you suspect you have a digestive enzyme deficiency, bitter herbs are the next step in repairing your digestion. Apple cider vinegar is acidic and works to replace stomach acid, but this is a Band-Aid solution. We want to stimulate your stomach to produce sufficient amounts of acid. The same principle applies to digestive enzymes. Supplementing with digestive enzymes is also a Band-Aid solution and is not making your body do what it should normally be doing. There are some instances where using digestive enzymes is helpful, but they should not be used widely by the general population to fix digestive concerns.

Bitter herbs are exactly what the name implies. They are herbs that taste bitter and stimulate the body to produce and release appropriate amounts of stomach acid, digestive enzymes, and bile to digest food.[129] They do taste awful, but they work incredibly well. Bitter herbs come in tincture form, and the strength of the product you use will determine the dose. Follow the label instructions for the product you are using. I recommend using bitter herbs at low doses immediately before every meal for two to three months. Possible adverse effects of bitter herbs include stomach upset, constipation, and increased sensitivity to sunlight.[130-142] Once the treatment course is over, discontinue the bitter herbs and pay attention to your digestion. Most of the time, patients are feeling much better, and we can move on to the next step. If any symptoms are lingering, we may need to correct other imbalances before moving on.

Note: There are a number of conditions in which bitter herbs should not be used. Bitter herbs should not be used if you have gallstones, kidney stones, gastritis, a peptic ulcer, or a history of an ulcer in the past.[129]

## Probiotics

Probiotics are bacteria contained in a pill or liquid form intended to contribute to a healthy population of bacteria in our intestines. I don't generally recommend probiotics to many of my fibromyalgia patients until we have determined that they do not have small intestinal bacterial overgrowth (SIBO), since taking a probiotic when you have SIBO can make you feel much worse. If you have been investigated for SIBO and do not have it, a probiotic is a reasonable addition to your digestion repair plan. When selecting a probiotic, opt for a product that has multiple strains of *Lactobacillus* and *Bifidobacterium* in it. Dosing of probiotics varies widely. A total dose of 10–20 billion CFU per day is sufficient. Possible adverse effects from the use of probiotics include stomach upset, bloating, and flatulence.[134-135]

At times, it is not the probiotic itself that people don't tolerate but the fructooligosaccharides (FOS) used in the supplement to keep the bacteria alive. It is possible to find capsule forms of probiotics that do not contain FOS, but it can be challenging. An alternative is to consume foods containing probiotics, which include kombucha, kefir, sauerkraut, tempeh, miso, and kimchi, at least two to three times per week.

Note: Probiotics should not be used if you have a diagnosed immunodeficiency condition.

## L-Glutamine

L-glutamine is my top choice for healing the gut lining. Glutamine is an amino acid that is made within the body.[136] Our need for glutamine increases substantially when we are under stress. In terms of repairing the digestive tract, glutamine acts as food for the cells lining our gut. When these cells are fed and well-nourished, they gradually grow back towards each other and repair any leaky holes in the gut lining. Without any leaking of the gut lining, inflammation levels decrease, and symptoms resolve.

The healing process takes some time, and I generally recommend taking L-glutamine at a dose of 5–10 grams per day for three months. Most L-glutamine supplements come in a powder form that is easily dissolved into water. Possible adverse effects from L-glutamine supplementation include nausea, fatigue, and muscle pain.[136] I have had some of my more sensitive patients react poorly to L-glutamine. It's not common, but it does happen. If that's the case, see the *Demulcent Herbs* section for an alternative gut-healing option.

## Demulcent Herbs

A *demulcent herb* is one that soothes irritated and inflamed tissues.[129] Demulcent herbs have many uses, one of which is healing the gut lining in instances of leaky gut or ulcerative diseases. Under normal conditions, the gut lining produces mucus to protect the cells from damage by stomach acid and digestive enzymes. If we didn't have this mucus layer, the acid and enzymes would digest our own lining, which would not be good. These herbs work to protect the lining of the gut by increasing the amount of protective mucus produced by the cells. This provides a thicker barrier between the cells and the acids and enzymes.[129]

There are a number of demulcent herbs that can be used to heal the gut lining. Examples include marshmallow (*Althea officinalis*), oats (*Avena sativa*), flax (*Linum usitatissimum*), licorice (*Glycyrrhiza glabra*), meadowsweet (*Filipendula ulmaria*), and slippery elm (*Ulmus rubra*).[129] These herbs work best as a tea or in food form in the case of oats and flax. When prepared properly, the tea will have a slippery, gummy texture.[129] Demulcent herbs are well tolerated overall, but as with anything taken orally, there is a risk of digestive upset. The herbs listed above can be used alone or in combination and can be found through various supplement and tea companies. Typical dosing of demulcent herbs is dependent on the product. Daily consumption for three months is generally required to repair the gut lining.

## KEY POINTS

- There are several common roadblocks to optimal digestion, including intestinal hyperpermeability (also known as leaky gut), hypochlorhydria, and digestive enzyme deficiency.
- If you've reacted to foods on the elimination diet, you likely have intestinal hyperpermeability.
- Do the Apple Cider Vinegar Challenge to determine if your stomach acid is low.
- Bitter herbs will correct low stomach acid levels and digestive enzyme deficiencies.
- L-glutamine helps heal the gut lining if you are experiencing intestinal hyperpermeability.
- If L-glutamine is not tolerated, demulcent herbs are another option for healing the gut lining.
- Probiotics can be added if you are sure you don't have SIBO.

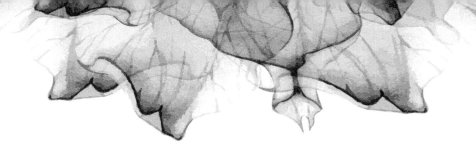

# CHAPTER 11

# RESTORE MITOCHONDRIAL FUNCTION

## WHAT ARE MITOCHONDRIA AND WHY ARE THEY IMPORTANT?

With optimal digestion in place, it's now time to address energy production in the mitochondria. To recap what we discussed in Chapter 2, the mitochondria are responsible for producing the energy that our cells need to carry out necessary functions and survive. Within the mitochondria, a number of chemical reactions occur to produce this energy in the form of ATP. Without ATP, our cells would not be able to carry out the processes that keep us alive, including breathing, digesting food and absorbing nutrients, moving our muscles, processing thoughts with our brains, etc. Almost everything our bodies do is dependent on ATP in some way.

As was also mentioned in Chapter 2, there are several issues with mitochondria in the cells of people with fibromyalgia. Dysfunction of the mitochondria leads to decreased amounts of ATP, which prevents cells from functioning properly and manifests as symptoms.[11,13-17] In the mitochondria of someone with fibromyalgia, several important enzymes don't function properly. Because of these defective enzymes the body destroys the mitochondria, leading to fewer mitochondria in people with fibromyalgia compared to people without fibromyalgia.[11,14-16] Unfortunately, this cycle is repeated when the body replaces the destroyed mitochondria with new mitochondria that also don't function well. Additionally, there are deficiencies in key nutrients required for the mitochondria to function.[11,14-16] The good news is that when nutrients are replenished and the mitochondria have what they need, mitochondrial function and fibromyalgia symptoms improve.[15]

The foundations of healing discussed in Chapter 6 are just as important here in addressing mitochondrial function as they are in supporting any other aspect of your health. If you're feeling fuzzy on what the foundations of health were, go back and review them. They will be essential to repairing and supporting your mitochondria and setting the stage for the supplemental options we will discuss next.

## SUPPLEMENTAL MITOCHONDRIAL SUPPORT

### When to Choose Which Form of Mitochondrial Support

There are a number of options for mitochondrial support. It can be tricky to know which to choose, and it may require some trial and error to find what works for you. Where applicable, I have included some tips based on my clinical experience. Potential medication interactions with specific supplements should also be a consideration in this choice.

Where possible and safe, I often use a supplement that is a combination of coenzyme Q10, acetyl-L-carnitine, and alpha-lipoic acid. I find that this combination can help decrease the number of pills required to effectively reduce pain, fatigue, and brain fog. Not everyone reacts well to this combination, and it is impossible to know which ingredient they do not respond well to without trying each individually. If you are not getting appropriate symptom relief with one mitochondrial support agent, it may be worthwhile to add a second, depending on the symptoms you are experiencing. Unless using a combination product, I recommend starting each supplement separately to save you money and allow you to determine what is working and/or causing adverse effects, if applicable.

## Coenzyme Q10 (CoQ10)

Coenzyme Q10 (CoQ10) is considered a *vitamin-like compound* that functions as an antioxidant and a participant in energy-generating pathways, particularly within the mitochondria.[137] The term *vitamin-like compound* means that CoQ10 acts similarly to vitamins but is produced in sufficient amounts within the body and so is not considered essential.[138] This means that CoQ10 is hugely important, but under normal circumstances the body can produce what it needs for metabolic processes.[137] CoQ10 is produced within the body from a number of nutrients, including various B vitamins, vitamin C, and minerals.[137] It is possible for CoQ10 to be deficient because of deficiencies in these nutrients.[137]

In the context of using CoQ10 to treat fibromyalgia, studies show that taking 300mg of CoQ10 daily for three months reduces pain, improves energy, and reduces sleep disturbances by about 20%–30% compared to fibromyalgia patients who did not receive CoQ10.[139-140] Some studies have even shown an improvement in mood with CoQ10 supplementation, specifically in decreased symptoms of depression.[141-142] CoQ10 is also an effective treatment option for those who experience migraines and headaches. Supplementation with CoQ10 has significantly decreased the incidence and severity of headaches in people with fibromyalgia.[142]

In fibromyalgia, CoQ10 as a treatment on its own is useful when pain and fatigue are the most debilitating symptoms. It is less helpful when brain fog is the predominant symptom in the fibromyalgia picture. Since CoQ10 is also very helpful in reducing the frequency and intensity of headaches and migraines, it would be my top choice for mitochondrial support for fibromyalgia with accompanying migraines.[137]

Typical doses of CoQ10 range from 300–400mg in three divided doses daily.[139-142] CoQ10 should be taken with food and in the earlier part of the day. Some people notice a significant energy boost with CoQ10, which can disrupt sleep if taken too close to bedtime. CoQ10 supplementation is generally well tolerated, but possible adverse effects include nausea, diarrhea, heartburn, decreased appetite, and abdominal discomfort.[137] CoQ10 can lower blood pressure slightly and may cause symptoms in people who have low blood pressure. Symptoms related to low blood pressure could include dizziness, light-headedness, fainting, blurred vision, nausea, fatigue, or lack of concentration.[143] Since CoQ10 can decrease blood pressure, it is ideal to have blood pressure measured prior to starting supplementation and monitored throughout treatment. Typically, blood pressure decreases are not an issue, but some people with fibromyalgia already suffer from symptomatic low blood pressure. If this is the case, start at a low dose and monitor blood pressure more frequently.

## Acetyl-L-Carnitine

Acetyl-L-carnitine is an amino acid that is made within the human body from other amino acids. It works within the mitochondria in the metabolic process of turning fat into ATP for cell use.[144] Without appropriate carnitine levels, mitochondria cannot function normally. Carnitine has also been shown to affect gene expression and nerve function.[144] It also appears to improve mood and cognitive function, especially in the areas of memory, attention, and cognitive fatigue.[144]

In studies performed in people with fibromyalgia, doses of 500mg three times per day, for a total of 1500mg daily, has been used for 8–12 weeks.[145-146] Carnitine supplementation can help reduce pain and improve depression symptoms, as well as improve ratings of quality of life.[145-146] Possible adverse effects of supplementation with acetyl-L-carnitine include nausea, vomiting, stomach upset, decreased appetite, headache, and insomnia.[144] To minimize the possibility of digestive adverse effects, take acetyl-L-carnitine with food and earlier in the day where possible.

Fiona had been diagnosed with fibromyalgia before her most recent car accident and felt as though she couldn't fully recover from this one. She had made progress with her fibromyalgia symptoms in the past and had been feeling good. Since the accident, however, she was having difficulty with her memory and processing information. She was also struggling with regulating her sleep and had to nap several times per day. We had already tried several treatment options to get Fiona back on track, but she wasn't responding to anything. I recommended she try acetyl-L-carnitine, starting at a moderate dose to see how she felt. When I saw Fiona a week later, she couldn't believe how much energy she had. She felt like she'd been struck by lightning and had to keep moving. She even had a dance party in her living room! While she loved this high energy, she still couldn't get her sleep schedule back to normal. We decreased her dose slightly and shifted the dose to earlier in the morning, so it would not disrupt her sleep.

Despite the limited amount of research available for use in fibromyalgia, acetyl-L-carnitine works well in relieving specific symptoms. Clinically, I use acetyl-L-carnitine when brain fog and memory difficulty are the main life-disrupting symptoms of fibromyalgia. It is less effective for pain relief. I have found acetyl-L-carnitine to be highly effective in increasing energy levels, so much so that caution must be taken to avoid disrupting sleep. If you experience an energy boost with acetyl-L-carnitine supplementation, ensure you are taking it earlier in the day to avoid sleep disruption.

Note: Acetyl-L-carnitine is a specific form of L-carnitine. There are other forms, but acetyl-L-carnitine is the form that has been studied in fibromyalgia.

## Alpha-Lipoic Acid

Alpha-lipoic acid (often abbreviated ALA) is an antioxidant that is made within the body. As an antioxidant, it has an anti-inflammatory effect on a number of tissues, including the blood vessels and nerves.[147] Alpha-lipoic acid also functions in the metabolism of carbohydrates to energy and in the mitochondria to assist in ATP production.[147] Since alpha-lipoic acid has a role in mitochondrial function and is used effectively in the treatment of neuropathic pain, there has been interest in it as a possible treatment option for fibromyalgia.[147-149] Although studies on alpha-lipoic acid use specifically in fibromyalgia are ongoing, it can be a useful adjunct to mitochondrial support and relief of nerve pain.

Dosing in fibromyalgia specifically has not been established, but typical doses of alpha-lipoic acid range from 600–1800mg daily.[147] Generally, alpha-lipoic acid is well tolerated. Possible adverse effects include nausea or vomiting.[147] To avoid digestive upset, take alpha-lipoic acid with food. Alpha-lipoic acid does not have the same effect on energy levels as acetyl-L-carnitine or coenzyme Q10 and can be taken at any time of day.

Alpha-lipoic acid can be very helpful in relieving pain but has little effect on the other symptoms of fibromyalgia, such as brain fog and fatigue. I find alpha-lipoic acid particularly effective for pain that is related to nerves, rather than pain associated with muscle tension. Nerve pain is typically sharp or shooting in nature. It may travel from one area of the body to another and can feel like an electric shock. When nerves are affected, symptoms can also include numbness or tingling. This is the type of pain that alpha-lipoic acid is more likely to be effective in relieving.

## D-Ribose

D-ribose is a sugar that is used in the structural formation of DNA, ATP, and enzymes that play a role in the mitochondrial energy-generating pathways.[150] It has been shown to improve energy and sleep, as well as reduce pain in people with fibromyalgia.[151] Additionally, D-ribose has been used to assist with muscle recovery and exercise tolerance in other patient populations.[152] Clinically, results with D-ribose can be inconsistent, but some people with fibromyalgia do experience benefit. I find this supplement particularly helpful when there is significant fatigue or pain after exercise, when starting a new exercise regimen, or when increasing exercise. D-ribose does not have an effect on brain fog. Outside of its relation to exercise, I do not typically use D-ribose for pain and fatigue due to inconsistency in results.

When adding D-ribose to a supplement regimen, dosing is typically five grams of D-ribose three times per day.[150] Most D-ribose supplements come as a powder that is mixed into a beverage and consumed. It does not matter whether D-ribose is taken with food or not. Most people tolerate supplementation at any time of day. Possible adverse effects of D-ribose supplementation include low blood sugar, stomach upset, headache, and decreased appetite.[150]

## KEY POINTS

- Mitochondrial support will further decrease pain, fatigue, and brain fog symptoms.
- CoQ10 is most helpful for pain, fatigue, and depression.
- CoQ10 is also effective for reducing migraines and headaches.
- Acetyl-L-carnitine is useful for pain, fatigue, brain fog, and memory difficulties.
- Alpha-lipoic acid can be added to other mitochondrial supports or used alone for nerve pain.
- D-ribose is most helpful when beginning an exercise regimen, increasing the intensity of exercise, or when pain and fatigue after exercise are the main concerns.
- Where possible, choose a product containing a combination of CoQ10, acetyl-L-carnitine, and alpha-lipoic acid.

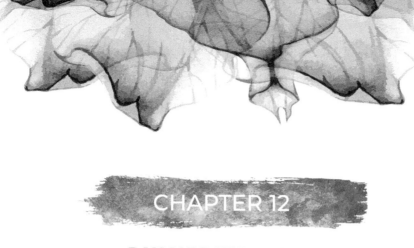

# CHAPTER 12

# PULVERIZE PAIN

Most often, once you've reached this stage of your health journey, pain levels are much lower than they were before. This chapter can be useful when you are still figuring out other parts of your overall health regimen, such as which diet, sleep, and mitochondrial supports work for you. It can also be useful as a resource when you are in a period of stress. With fibromyalgia, pain can flare when experiencing higher than normal stress, despite your dedication to continuing with the healthy habits and supplements that have worked for you previously.

There are times when pain is what we need to address early on in a treatment plan, because it is the one symptom that is preventing you from functioning and having the motivation to implement other changes to improve your health. There's nothing wrong with that. Be mindful that the strategies presented prior to this section will also help bring down pain levels. If you use the strategies discussed in this chapter first, be aware that it may be more difficult to see how much other health changes are helping, unless you wait until your pain levels have reached a new consistent level before starting anything else.

I have divided this chapter into strategies for fast pain relief and options that provide longer-term pain relief. The fast pain relief options will be helpful when you are in a flare or having a bad day. The longer-term pain relief strategies are for pain that is consistently present. These strategies will not help with pain in the moment and require consistent use to see benefit.

## FAST PAIN RELIEF

### Hydrotherapy

While hydrotherapy is not a supplement, it can be very effective for pain relief in fibromyalgia.[160–161] At times, hydrotherapy can be more effective than supplement options. Hydrotherapy is the use of water at different temperatures to bring about change within the body. On initial exposure to cold water, blood flow to an area decreases; however, blood flow increases with longer exposure and after exposure to warm the area. Hot water increases blood flow to a specific area. Used together and in an alternating fashion, the temperature contrast can increase blood flow, warm the body, boost the immune system, and increase energy levels.

Most people have a preference for which temperature they find relieves their pain. Whether it's hot or cold, if you find that one makes a difference for you, use this to your advantage. Using hydrotherapy can help dull pain and increase energy, while preventing you from having to take another pill.

There are a number of different ways you can use hydrotherapy. The practices I recommend most frequently to my patients are contrast showers, infrared sauna sessions, and Epsom salt baths. You must have access to an infrared sauna for the second to be an option for you. Some can access this at home or at the gym. Some people feel light-headed and dizzy during or after using these methods. For your safety, please be sure you have someone with you the first few times you try hydrotherapy. See the *Additional Resources* section for instructions on how to implement the hydrotherapy techniques discussed here.

### Contrast Showers

Contrast showers involve an alternation between hot and cold water during a regular shower. You want to start with hot water and then switch to cold water. A time ratio of 3:1 works well. For example, three minutes of hot water and then one minute of cold water, or 1.5 minutes of hot water and 30 seconds of cold water. You will want to include three to five cycles (one cycle is hot then cold) in one session, always finishing with cold water. The greater the temperature difference between hot and cold, the more pronounced the effects will be. It is a good idea to start with smaller temperature differences to determine how you respond to contrast showers, before moving on to larger temperature differences.

My patient Beth refers to contrast showers as a "special kind of torture." She hates the idea of doing them, especially in the winter, but if she doesn't do them, she craves them. Beth tends to feel cold often, which brings on her pain and decreases her energy. When Beth started doing contrast showers, she noticed how much warmer she felt throughout the day. Her hands and feet wouldn't get as cold, and she experienced much less muscle pain. Beth does contrast showers on days when she has more activities planned, since she gets an energy boost for a few hours afterward.

## Infrared Sauna Sessions

Sauna therapy can be used to encourage detoxification, relieve pain, and improve energy levels. As mentioned previously, you must have access to a sauna for this to be an option for you. To improve your tolerance for sauna therapy, ensure you are drinking enough water throughout the session. Electrolyte water is the preferred form of hydration to replace electrolytes lost to sweating. Sauna sessions can be included in pain management strategies up to five times weekly, with most patients responding well to three sessions weekly for 30–60 minutes. If possible, start at a lower temperature to determine how you tolerate saunas.

## Epsom Salt Baths

Epsom salts are made of magnesium sulphate and dissolve easily into warm bath water. When you soak in a warm Epsom salt bath, the pores on your skin open, allowing the magnesium to be absorbed. As described previously, magnesium has a variety of benefits in fibromyalgia. The use of Epsom salts specifically benefits pain levels and muscle tension. If you enjoy baths, it is also a great form of stress management and relaxation therapy. To get the pain-relieving benefits of Epsom salts, add one to two cups of Epsom salts to the desired temperature of bath water and soak for at least 20 minutes as often as daily.

## Topical Pain Relief

There are a number of topical options that can be used to help with pain relief. I have outlined several below. Since these are intended for topical use only, please do not take internally. Possible adverse effects with these pain-relieving methods include skin irritation, itching, or rash. If you notice any adverse effects, discontinue immediately. Topical options minimize the risk of medication interactions, unless your medication is also applied topically.

*Castor Oil*

Castor oil is an anti-inflammatory oil that can be applied topically for pain relief and inflammation control. Castor oil is a thick, clear oil that is absorbed into the skin over time. I recommend castor oil to my patients for joint and muscle pain, as well as arthritic conditions. See the *Additional Resources* section for instructions on how to apply castor oil.

*LivRelief*

LivRelief is an over-the-counter cream containing a mixture of herbs that help relieve pain and inflammation. This cream can be applied topically one to two times per day. Pain relief with LivRelief is fast and can be enough to take the edge off. LivRelief is widely available at most pharmacies.

*Arnica Cream*

Arnica can be used in herbal form and homeopathic form. Topical versions of arnica cream can be applied to the painful area daily. Arnica cream is inexpensive and can bring about pain relief quickly.

# LONG-TERM PAIN RELIEF

## Magnesium

Magnesium is highly effective for pain management in fibromyalgia. See Chapter 9 for more information.

## Palmitoylethanolamide (PEA)

Palmitoylethanolamide (PEA) is a fatty acid that is made naturally by the body in response to stress and pain.[153] There has been interest in using PEA as a treatment in conditions related to brain inflammation.[154] If you recall from Chapter 2, inflammation within the brain has been identified as a possible contributor to fibromyalgia development.[8,31]

PEA has been shown to reduce pain in a number of chronic pain conditions, including fibromyalgia.[154–158] Research also suggests that PEA may have a role in decreasing intestinal permeability and gut healing.[153] In people with fibromyalgia, supplementation with PEA appears to reduce pain and improve scores on the fibromyalgia impact questionnaire.[157–158] More research is needed to determine the full effects of PEA in fibromyalgia.

Doses of PEA typically range between 600–1200mg for the treatment of fibromyalgia.[153] There are no known drug interactions between PEA and medications. Adverse effects from supplementation tend to be minimal, but could include nausea, diarrhea, bloating, constipation, vomiting, palpitations, and dizziness.[153,157]

## Curcumin

Curcumin is another name for the spice turmeric. It can be used in food and as a supplement for its potent anti-inflammatory properties. Curcumin can be used as a pain reliever and has been researched for joint pain due to arthritis and painful periods.[159] While curcumin has not been studied in fibromyalgia, it is commonly used among patients and practitioners. Given the evidence showing brain inflammation and symptoms related to digestive inflammation in fibromyalgia, curcumin is a logical treatment choice.

Curcumin doses range widely, from 180mg to over 2 grams per day. Doses used for painful conditions typically range from 1–2 grams (1000–2000mg) per day.[159] Curcumin should always be taken with food to assist with absorption and prevent digestion-related adverse effects. Possible adverse effects include constipation, stomach upset, diarrhea, bloating, heartburn, nausea, and vomiting.[159] Many people experience pain relief within the first two weeks of curcumin supplementation; however, its full effects may not be apparent until after two to three months of supplementation.

## Boswellia

Boswellia is another anti-inflammatory herb that is often used for arthritis conditions, such as unspecified joint pain, osteoarthritis, and rheumatoid arthritis.[162] Although it has not been specifically studied in people with fibromyalgia, it can bring pain relief to some. Boswellia is more useful in people with fibromyalgia who experience pain that is more localized to joints, rather than generalized muscle pain. In diagnosed arthritis conditions, boswellia reduces inflammation and relieves pain.[162]

Doses of boswellia range from 100–250 mg daily.[162] Boswellia is best absorbed when taken with a meal containing fat.[162] Possible adverse effects of boswellia supplementation include diarrhea, nausea, abdominal pain, heartburn, itching, headache, swelling, and general weakness.[162]

## Devil's Claw

Devil's claw is an herb that is often used for painful conditions, including low back pain, osteoarthritis, rheumatoid arthritis, and fibromyalgia.[163] It has not been specifically studied in fibromyalgia but can be used when inflammation is suspected to be contributing to pain.

Dosing of devil's claw is typically in the range of 2000–2400mg daily, in divided doses with food. The possibility of diarrhea is the most common adverse effect from devil's claw supplementation but only affects about 8% of people who use it.[163]

Note: Anti-inflammatory herbs can be combined and may be more effective for pain relief in combinations, rather than on their own.

## WHEN TO CHOOSE WHICH OPTION

Not all of these methods work for everyone. It will take some time to find what works best for you. Beyond modulating sleep and mitochondrial support, there is little research in the area of pain control in fibromyalgia. Some of these supplements are used because they are effective in other painful conditions or because they reduce inflammation, which has been shown to be a contributor to fibromyalgia. Other options provide fast pain relief when you are in a flare or having a bad day. I have listed the options here in the order in which I would use them, assuming that they are all possibilities in terms of safety and medication interactions. Always check with your health care provider to determine whether a new supplement is safe for you. As mentioned previously, anti-inflammatory and pain-relieving herbs can often be combined to achieve better pain control.

## KEY POINTS

- Fast pain relief strategies are useful during a flare or when having a bad day.
- Hydrotherapy is a great option for pain relief and can include contrast showers, infrared sauna sessions, and Epsom salt baths.
- Topical pain relief options include castor oil, LivRelief, or arnica cream.
- Longer-term pain relief strategies will provide pain relief over time, but not immediately.
- Longer-term pain relief options need to be used consistently to see a benefit in pain levels.
- Magnesium and palmitoylethanolamide have been studied in fibromyalgia and show benefit for pain relief.
- Other longer-term pain relief options include curcumin, boswellia, and devil's claw.

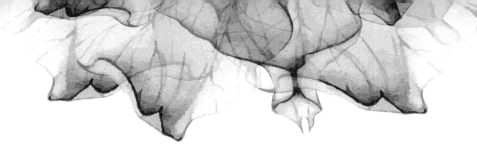

# CHAPTER 13

# BALANCING THE STRESS RESPONSE

Now that you have strategies to manage any existing pain and address it when it flares, we want to focus on retraining your body to respond to stress properly. Stress comes in many forms and includes any event or situation that requires a reaction from your body.[164] Examples include a change in environmental temperature, injury, illness, infection, exposure to toxins, or an emotional reaction.[164] Our bodies respond to all types of stressors in the same way, meaning that physiologically we cannot distinguish between emotional and physical stressors. The stress response is always the same. Even happy emotional events are a form of stress to the body. For example, think of how tired you may feel after celebrating the marriage of someone close to you.

Stress is not inherently a bad thing and is an unavoidable part of normal, everyday life. The key to how stress affects us is how we respond to it. As mentioned previously, the stress response is dysfunctional in fibromyalgia and does not shut off when it should. So, what does a normal stress response look like? Stress researcher Hans Selye developed the theory of *general adaptation syndrome* to describe how the body normally responds to stress.[164]

## GENERAL ADAPTATION SYNDROME

According to the theory of general adaptation syndrome, the body's stress response has three phases: alarm, resistance, and exhaustion.[164] Although these phases sound separate, in truth they are a continuum. All three phases are largely controlled by the adrenal glands, which sit on top of the kidney like little hats and release hormones that regulate stress and other bodily functions.[164]

### Alarm Phase

The alarm phase is the body's initial response to stress. A stressful event occurs, and the sympathetic nervous system is activated. Recall from Chapter 6 that the sympathetic nervous system is responsible for fight-or-flight changes in the body. Stress hormone release is regulated by the hypothalamic–pituitary–adrenal (HPA) axis. The hypothalamus and pituitary gland are parts of the brain that receive messages from the body and send messages to the adrenal glands (among other body parts) to regulate hormonal release.

When the sympathetic nervous system and the HPA axis are active in the initial phase of the stress response, adrenaline is released from the adrenal glands. This causes changes within the body that allow appropriate responses to whatever danger has been perceived. These changes include increased heart rate and stronger contraction by the heart muscle, increased blood flow to the brain, heart, and muscles (and consequently away from reproductive and digestive organs), increased respiratory rate to supply the cells with adequate oxygen, increased sweat production, and increased blood sugar levels to provide the cells with adequate energy.[164] Ideally, the stressful event is short, and the body can then return to its normal state, shutting off the fight-or-flight reaction. Your experience of the alarm phase may include feeling high-strung, anxious or agitated. Your blood pressure and heart rate may stay within the normal range or increase.

## Resistance Phase

When there are a number of ongoing or sequential stressors, the body moves from alarm phase into resistance phase.[164] In the resistance phase, the body continues to respond to the stressor and mobilize appropriate resources to cope with this perceived danger after the initial fight-or-flight response has subsided. In the resistance phase, cortisol is released from the adrenal glands.[164] Cortisol is the hormone we typically classify as our stress hormone. Most often, glucose stores are used up in the alarm phase. This means that another source of energy must be found to supply energy to active cells in the resistance phase. Protein is typically the source of energy used in this phase.[164] Protein may be obtained from the diet or by breaking down muscle and organ tissue. Continued exposure to high stress and maintenance of the resistance phase results in tissue damage, increases the risk of disease, and eventually leads to the third phase, exhaustion.[164] Your experience of the resistance phase may include feeling anxious, irritable, depressed, driven, and overreactive. Often, you are working to compensate for fatigue in this stage. Blood pressure and heart rate are either normal or high in this stage.

## Exhaustion Phase

The exhaustion phase is also known as burnout. Because of the long-term continuation of the stress response, the body does not have the ability to repair damaged tissues and achieve balance in metabolic processes. Organ systems and bodily functions may weaken or begin to shut down.[164] The adrenal glands cannot continue producing high levels of cortisol, and we see low cortisol levels in this phase of general adaptation syndrome. Recovery from this phase can be a lengthy process and requires significant tissue healing. Your experience of the exhaustion phase may include extreme fatigue, inability to tolerate even mild to moderate stress, anxiety, depression, and irritability. In this stage, blood pressure and heart rate are low and can be difficult to increase.

## THE STRESS RESPONSE AND FIBROMYALGIA

With fibromyalgia, we see signs that the body is not functioning optimally. Research shows that there is evidence of dysfunction in muscle structure and function, mitochondrial dysfunction, immune dysfunction, and brain inflammation, as described in Chapter 2.[11–16,18–21,29–31] Physiologically, this translates to a system that is on high alert for danger. This is a system that is using up all of its resources to maintain a stress response that will not shut off. This disrupts cortisol balance, sleep, and gut bacteria and results in nutrient deficiencies.[22–28,32–36]

I've seen fibromyalgia patients in all stages of general adaptation syndrome. Some have recently experienced a major stressor and are in the alarm phase. Others have reached the resistance phase, and still others have reached burnout. It is ideal if we can prevent the exhaustion phase, but all hope is not lost if that's where you suspect you are.

Whether we can change the amount of stress you're under or not, we can change the way you respond to stress in the future. I urge you to work on reducing your exposure to stressors as much as possible and training your body to enter a state of calm more frequently, but as we know, some stress in life is inevitable. This chapter includes supplemental and herbal options for supporting your body during stressful periods of your life or while working on reducing your exposure to stress and managing your reaction to it.

## ADAPTOGENS

Adaptogens are herbs that increase the body's tolerance to stress and allow the body to experience stress for longer periods before reaching burnout.[165] We use adaptogens to decrease the initial stress response, prolong the resistance phase, and protect the body from exposure to long-term stress.[165] Different adaptogens will have different effects on the body and may be more useful in some stages of the stress response than others. There are many herbs that act as adaptogens, and I've included only the ones I use most frequently in the treatment of fibromyalgia here. Very few of these herbs have been specifically researched as a treatment for fibromyalgia; however, they are commonly used by patients and practitioners alike.

### Non-Stimulating Adaptogens

Adaptogens classified as non-stimulating are my ideal choice for use in people with fibromyalgia. Because people with fibromyalgia tend to be sensitive to supplements, the addition of a stimulating herb can cause more problems than it solves. The use of a stimulating herb can result in overuse of energy and the beginnings of a crash cycle.

It can decrease the amount of deep sleep you are getting and negate any progress made in regulating sleep. Non-stimulating adaptogens have the benefit of managing the stress response and supporting the immune system without overstimulation. These adaptogens prevent damage to body tissues and stabilize energy levels, without providing false energy.

*Holy Basil*

Holy basil is a wonderfully calming and gentle adaptogen. It can be used to calm the body's stress response when there is significant anxiety and sleep dysfunction occurring.[166] Holy basil can help minimize the tissue damage that long-term stress can cause.[165] For this reason, it is considered a *building adaptogen*, meaning that it helps to build the body up. In contrast to licorice, which is described later in this chapter, holy basil helps lower cortisol levels when they are high.[165] This can help prevent the detrimental effects of high stress on body tissues and slow the progression to the exhaustion phase. Holy basil has been shown to balance blood sugar levels, protect against inflammation, and balance the immune response.[165]

In addition to use during stress, holy basil is useful in addressing brain fog and poor memory.[165] I also use holy basil when there has been a significant trauma that a patient is having trouble processing or is receiving counselling for, as it can be helpful in addressing depression.[165] Since holy basil is gentle and has a host of additional benefits that are helpful in fibromyalgia, it is one of my top choices for my fibromyalgia patients.

Holy basil is most often found in capsule form but can also be found in tincture or tea form. In tea form, it is often called tulsi. Dosing of holy basil in capsule form ranges from 400mg to 2.5 grams daily at any time of day.[166] Possible adverse effects from holy basil include nausea and loose stools.[166] These effects can be minimized by taking holy basil with food.

### Rhodiola

Rhodiola does not give the sensation of an energy boost but does allow the body to function better when under stress. This effect is seen in studies on rhodiola supplementation as increased time to fatigue, increased ability to handle a larger workload, improved energy ratings, and improved memory and concentration, as well as improved mood.[167] In addition to its adaptogenic properties, rhodiola can be used to treat anxiety, depression, and insomnia.[167] In fibromyalgia, I choose rhodiola when there are mood concerns such as anxiety or depression and when poor memory or focus are present.

Rhodiola is most commonly found in capsule form but can also be used in tincture or tea form. Doses of rhodiola in capsule form range from 170–680mg daily.[167] Adverse effects from the use of rhodiola are typically mild, but could include dizziness and change in saliva production (increase or decrease).[167] If taking rhodiola, it is ideal to take it earlier in the day (mid-afternoon or before), without food where possible.

### Ashwagandha

Ashwagandha (also known as withania) is similar to holy basil but is slightly more stimulating and has more targeted effects on the immune system. In research performed on people under stress, ashwagandha was shown to reduce levels of perceived stress by 33%–44% and lower cortisol levels by 22%–28%, compared to treatment with a placebo.[168] Use of ashwagandha can also help lower anxiety levels, improve memory and cognition, modulate the immune system, and reduce inflammation.[168] In some studies, ashwagandha has also been shown to have a pain-relieving effect.[168]

I do not use ashwagandha as a treatment in fibromyalgia until we have determined whether the nightshade vegetables are a symptom trigger. For more information on how to determine symptom triggers, see Chapter 7. If nightshade vegetables are a trigger for pain, I avoid the use of ashwagandha because it is in the same family as the nightshade vegetables (the Solanaceae family).[168] If we have determined that the nightshade vegetables are not a trigger for pain, I may consider the use of ashwagandha. Since ashwagandha has been shown to help support thyroid function in hypothyroidism, I am more likely to choose it over other adaptogens if a patient has been diagnosed with both hypothyroidism and fibromyalgia.[168]

Similarly to the adaptogens we have already discussed, ashwagandha is available in capsule, tea, or tincture form. It is also commonly available in powder form. Dosing in capsule form typically ranges from 250mg to 5 grams daily.[168] Ashwagandha is usually well tolerated, but high doses can cause stomach upset, diarrhea, and vomiting.[168] Ashwagandha can be taken without food, but taking it with food can minimize these effects.

### Licorice

I would classify licorice as a non-stimulating adaptogen; however, licorice has a special effect in the body compared to other adaptogens. Licorice inhibits the enzyme in the body responsible for converting cortisol to its inactive form, cortisone.[169] This means that supplementation with licorice increases the length of time that cortisol is active within the body.[169] This effect is particularly helpful when cortisol levels are low or when exhaustion phase has been reached. Even with low cortisol production levels, increasing the amount of time that cortisol is active can improve symptoms significantly.

The component of licorice responsible for these adaptogenic effects is called glycyrrhizinic acid.[169] You can get licorice products containing glycyrrhizinic acid or with this component removed (called deglycyrrhizinated licorice, or DGL). Since DGL has had its glycyrrhizinic acid removed, it is not effective for use as an adaptogen.[169] It has other medical uses but will not help the body modulate the stress response.

Licorice is available in capsule form, as a tincture, or as a tea. It can be very effective in any of these forms. If you are particularly sensitive, it may be ideal to try a tea first, as this form tends to be the gentlest. Doses of licorice can range from 100mg to 2.5 grams daily.[169] Doses of licorice higher than 20 grams daily can be dangerous and should be avoided. If you are consuming multiple products containing licorice or eat licorice as a food, be sure to check your dose. The reason for this is that licorice raises blood pressure and can cause electrolyte imbalances, which can affect the functioning of the heart.[169] Blood pressure should always be measured prior to starting licorice and periodically afterwards. Avoid the use of licorice if you have high blood pressure, cardiovascular problems, or kidney conditions.[170] Possible adverse effects of licorice use include nausea, vomiting, or headaches.[169]

Note: Low blood pressure, also known as hypotension, is common in people with fibromyalgia. Licorice may be a great choice to minimize symptoms associated with low blood pressure, which can include dizziness, light-headedness, fainting, blurred vision, nausea, fatigue, or lack of concentration.[143]

## Stimulating Adaptogens

I rarely use stimulating adaptogens in the treatment of fibromyalgia, as described above. I find that the stimulating effect can make energy conservation difficult and result in further energy depletion. There have been cases where I use a stimulating adaptogen short term (for example, to assist a patient in getting through a specific event) and then switch back to a non-stimulating adaptogen. This is really the only scenario in which I recommend using stimulating adaptogens in fibromyalgia treatment.

*Panax Ginseng*

Panax ginseng is also known as Asian ginseng.[165] Since panax ginseng acts as a stimulant, it has been researched for its effects on fatigue, immunodeficiency, memory, and cognitive impairment, as well as athletic performance.[170] Panax ginseng has been shown to be beneficial in improving attention, reaction time, and performance of mental math in some populations but does not appear to have any benefit on memory.[170] Taking panax ginseng may help reduce physical fatigue ratings by about 66% and mental fatigue by about 50%, based on a study performed on people with fatigue of unknown cause.[170] In light of these improvements, it is not surprising that panax ginseng has been studied for use in fibromyalgia. In this study, a dose of 100mg daily of panax ginseng for 12 weeks did not improve pain, fatigue, sleep, anxiety, or number of tender points compared to a placebo.[171] The dose used in this fibromyalgia study was much lower than the dose of panax ginseng used in other studies, and this may have contributed to the lack of effect.

If a stimulating adaptogen is desired, panax ginseng may be a good option, but a dose higher than 100mg daily may be necessary, depending on tolerance. Doses of panax ginseng range from 100mg to 9 grams daily, with or without food. Possible adverse effects of panax ginseng use include insomnia, abnormal vaginal bleeding or loss of menses, blood pressure changes (increase or decrease), breast pain, water retention (edema), decreased appetite, diarrhea, itching, headache, vertigo, and mania.[170]

*Eleutherococcus*

Eleutherococcus also goes by the names of Siberian ginseng or eleuthero. It is another stimulating adaptogen that can be used to increase energy, improve cognitive performance, support athletic performance, and boost the immune system.[172] Eleutherococcus has not been studied in fibromyalgia specifically, but it has been studied in chronic fatigue syndrome, where research showed it had no effect on symptoms after two months of supplementation.[172] Research results on eleutherococcus and its effects on fatigue are less consistent than those of panax ginseng, with animal studies showing more benefit than human studies.[172] The adaptogenic effects of eleutherococcus are thought to be due to its ability to balance the HPA axis and cortisol levels.

In the treatment of fibromyalgia, I would only choose a stimulating adaptogen if there was a specific reason and timeframe for use. I would choose eleutherococcus over panax ginseng if panax ginseng was poorly tolerated, or there were concerns surrounding medication interactions or possible adverse effects. The possible adverse effects from eleutherococcus are far fewer and less severe than those associated with panax ginseng use.

Eleutherococcus is available in capsule form, as a tincture, or as a tea. Dosing of eleutherococcus typically ranges from 300–1200mg daily, apart from food.[172] Use of eleutherococcus for more than six weeks is generally not recommended.[172] Possible adverse effects of eleutherococcus include itching, hives, and skin rashes.[172] Clinically, I have also seen patients experience insomnia and agitation with use of eleutherococcus.

## OTHER HORMONAL IMBALANCES

Thyroid conditions and reproductive hormonal imbalances are also very common in people with fibromyalgia. While it is very important to address these imbalances and the symptoms they cause as well, it is not physically possible to include everything in this book. There are a number of wonderfully useful books written on these topics and many health care providers fluent in addressing these health concerns. When addressing other hormonal imbalances, the same dosing principles will apply. You will want to start with low doses of new supplements or medications and slowly increase the dose over time.

## KEY POINTS

- There are three phases to general adaptation syndrome: alarm phase, resistance phase, and exhaustion phase.
- With fibromyalgia, you can fall into any phase.
- Choose non-stimulating adaptogens over stimulating adaptogens.
- Only use stimulating adaptogens short term for a specific event or timeframe.
- Non-stimulating adaptogens include holy basil, rhodiola, ashwagandha, and licorice.
- Licorice is particularly useful in the exhaustion phase, as it increases the amount of time cortisol is active.
- Stimulating adaptogens include panax ginseng and eleutherococcus.

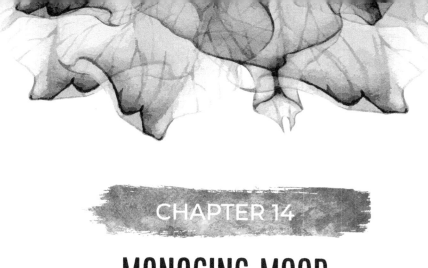

# CHAPTER 14

# MANAGING MOOD

Increasing your resilience to stress and retraining your body to respond appropriately will help with mood balance, but at times you may require additional mood support. Many people with fibromyalgia suffer from anxiety and depression as well. It is estimated that more than half of people with fibromyalgia will experience depression at some point in their lives. This number is much higher than what we see in the general population.[173] Unfortunately, depression and anxiety often go hand in hand with chronic pain conditions.[174]

Over the years, a number of theories have suggested that mood imbalances are the cause of fibromyalgia, but I strongly disagree. We have discussed the physiological abnormalities that occur in fibromyalgia, two of which are brain inflammation and an abnormal stress response. Both of these could be the root cause of the high rates of anxiety and depression in people with fibromyalgia. It is also very likely that the symptoms of fibromyalgia itself could contribute to increased anxiety and depression. Living with a condition that can be debilitating, unpredictable, and misunderstood by many and feeling sad or worried about it seems completely reasonable to me. Feeling sad and worried because your life is so different from how it used to be and how you imagined it would be also seems reasonable.

Regardless of why you're feeling sad or anxious, those feelings are valid. There are a number of ways to support mood balance naturally. We've already discussed important lifestyle practices, diet practices, digestion support, and natural ways to support a healthy stress response. All of the information discussed so far will be just as important for managing fibromyalgia symptoms as it is for supporting healthy mood balance.

## COUNSELLING

Since trauma is a common and prominent theme in the health history of many people with fibromyalgia, counselling may be a wonderful addition to the other health practices you've implemented so far.[7] Counselling is not an admission of defeat or a sign that you are broken. It is a courageous and intentional act of taking care of yourself and showing your mind, body, and spirit some much-needed love. When we have unprocessed or repressed emotions surrounding an event in our past or a current situation, we carry that around like a weight on our shoulders at all times. It manages to permeate everything we do and change the way we see and interact with the world. This is a big stressor for anyone. As we discussed in Chapter 13, our bodies physiologically respond to all forms of stress in the same way. This constant source of stress may be a major contributor to why your body can't shut off the stress response.

When seeking out a counsellor or mental health professional, be sure to choose one that is registered with a professional body. Typically, I refer to registered psychotherapists for high-quality mental health support; however, the title of the professional may differ depending on where you live. Within Canada, social workers, psychologists, and psychiatrists are also great options. When you choose a professional who is registered, you are choosing someone who is monitored by a regulatory body to ensure public safety, has a specific minimum amount of training, and is required to keep their training up-to-date with continuing education.

## NUTRIENTS

In Chapter 8 we discussed nutrient deficiencies, several of which can have depression as a symptom. If you are suffering from low mood, getting blood testing for deficiencies in iron, vitamin B12, and vitamin D is an important first step. Seek assistance from a health care provider for dosing of these nutrients, as they should be dosed based on a lab value.

## NATURE/EXERCISE

Spending time outside and in nature is one of the best mood boosters. It has been well documented that people who spend more time outside tend to be happier. If possible and your energy level allows, take a walk along a lake or in a forest. If engaging in exercise outside is not feasible for you, at least sit outside or relax near an open window as often as possible.

## SUPPLEMENTS FOR ANXIETY AND DEPRESSION

There are many natural treatment options available for addressing anxiety and depression. I have included the supplements I use most often here, but there are others. If your anxiety or depression is severe or you are experiencing suicidal thoughts, it is important that you speak with a health care provider, as these options may not be the best for you. It is also important to check with your health care provider if you are taking any medication, as some natural products can interact dangerously with medications used for anxiety and depression.

### L-Theanine

L-theanine is an effective and fast-acting treatment option for anxiety and worry.[123] It has also been used to treat depression;[123] however, I find it to be more effective for anxiety. L-theanine is found naturally in green tea and in some mushrooms.[123] We discussed L-theanine briefly in Chapter 9 as an option for sleep support. L-theanine helps improve sleep quality, particularly when anxiety and worry are the disruptors of sleep.[123]

L-theanine typically comes in chewable tablet form but can also be combined with other ingredients in capsule form. It can be taken daily or used on an as-needed basis for acute stress and anxiety. L-theanine is most commonly taken orally in doses of 100–200mg daily, with or without food.[123] Medication interactions and possible adverse effects are minimal with L-theanine. Possible adverse effects include headache or sleepiness.[123] Since L-theanine can be used to support sleep, it is best to try L-theanine in the evening initially to determine how you react to it.

## Passionflower

Although passionflower can be used to support sleep, I find it to be an effective anxiety-relieving herb that does not produce drowsiness in most users. It works quickly and can be used daily or as needed for anxiety symptoms. The anti-anxiety effects of passionflower have been compared to several anti-anxiety medications in research studies. In these studies, passionflower has been shown to be at least as effective as commonly used anxiety medications for relieving anxiety symptoms.[126] I find passionflower particularly effective in anxiety that can lead to panic attacks, as well as for addressing more severe daily anxiety.

Paula used to have panic attacks every time she was in a place with lots of people. She was embarrassed to go out in public and risk having a panic attack. She couldn't go to stores, social events, or put on presentations at work. Paula didn't want to have to take something every day if she didn't have to. I recommended that Paula take passionflower when she felt she needed it for symptoms of anxiety. Paula's first test of passionflower was going to a big family event. She took passionflower before the event and brought it with her in case she needed it. Paula did not experience any panic attacks at the family event, so she tried taking passionflower before running errands with her husband on a Saturday. She felt more anxious at the store but managed to complete her errands with no panic attacks. When the time came for Paula to give a presentation at work, she was ready to put the passionflower to the test. Presentations had always been the most anxiety-provoking events for Paula. With a quick dose of passionflower 30 minutes beforehand, Paula breezed through her presentation and finished feeling confident and excited.

Passionflower is available in capsule form and as a tincture or tea. Similar to L-theanine, it may be a good idea to initially try passionflower in the evening to determine how you respond to it. Doses of passionflower capsules range from 30–200mg daily.[126] Appropriate doses of tincture products depend on the strength of the product. Passionflower works better when taken apart from food. Possible adverse effects of passionflower use include dizziness, confusion, and sedation or sleepiness.[126]

## GABA

GABA (gamma-aminobutyric acid) is an inhibitory neurotransmitter that can be used to treat anxiety and stress. Similar to passionflower and L-theanine, GABA can be used as needed or on a daily basis. I typically use GABA in combination with L-theanine, as these two agents work well together. Research performed on GABA has shown that it helps relieve anxiety and increase concentration when performing a task.[175]

GABA is available in pill form, and doses typically range from 100mg to 2.5 grams daily, with or without food. Possible adverse effects include stomach upset, nausea, decreased appetite, constipation, or muscle weakness.[175] In some individuals, GABA can induce a sleepy feeling and may be used as a sleep aid. Initially, it is best to try GABA in the evening to determine how it affects you.

## 5-HTP

5-HTP was introduced previously in Chapter 9 as a sleep aid. To review, 5-HTP is produced from an amino acid called L-tryptophan and is used to make serotonin, which is a neurotransmitter involved in mood.[124] 5-HTP can be effective as a treatment option for both anxiety and depression.[124] Most studies on 5-HTP for depression have compared its effects to those of antidepressant medications. 5-HTP was shown to be as effective as several commonly used antidepressant medications in relieving depressive symptoms.[124] In treatment of anxiety, studies have shown that the addition of 5-HTP to some anti-anxiety medications decreased anxiety symptoms and phobias compared to the medication alone.[124]

Dosing of 5-HTP for the treatment of anxiety and depression ranges from 25–800mg daily. In research performed in people with fibromyalgia, 5-HTP at 100mg, three times per day for up to 90 days was studied. After 30 days on 5-HTP, people with fibromyalgia experienced improvements in number of tender points, intensity of pain, amount of sleep, anxiety, fatigue, and morning stiffness.[176] In another study, the same benefits were observed after only 15 days on 300mg daily of 5-HTP.[177] The results of this research suggest that 5-HTP may be helpful in reducing pain and tenderness and improving sleep, anxiety, and fatigue.[124,176-177] Possible adverse effects of 5-HTP use include nausea, vomiting, abdominal pain, diarrhea, and decreased appetite.[124] Taking 5-HTP with food typically minimizes digestive upset.

Since 5-HTP is the precursor to serotonin, it should not be taken alongside antidepressant medications. The combination of medications that alter serotonin levels and 5-HTP can cause a dangerous condition called serotonin syndrome, which can be fatal.[124] Be sure to check with your health care provider about any possible medication interactions prior to starting 5-HTP.

## SAMe

SAMe stands for S-adenosyl-L-methionine. It is a derivative of an amino acid and is used in the treatment of depression, anxiety, and fibromyalgia.[178] With respect to mood, SAMe has more research supporting its use in depression than in anxiety. Research performed on SAMe shows that it is at least as effective as tricyclic antidepressant medications, and some research shows that SAMe may be more effective.[178] Research performed on the use of 800mg daily of SAMe in fibromyalgia shows that SAMe can help improve symptoms of fibromyalgia, including pain, fatigue, morning stiffness, and mood within six weeks.[179]

Doses of SAMe range from 600–2400mg orally in divided doses daily.[178] It can take four to six weeks to see the full effects of SAMe on mood. In fibromyalgia, the dose studied was 400mg, twice per day for six weeks.[178] Possible adverse effects of SAMe use include flatulence, nausea, vomiting, diarrhea, constipation, dry mouth, headache, insomnia, reduced appetite, sweating, dizziness, and nervousness.[178] These adverse effects are more common at higher doses.[178] Similarly to 5-HTP, SAMe can affect serotonin levels and result in serotonin syndrome when combined with medications that alter serotonin levels.[178] Check with your health care provider to determine if SAMe is a safe option for you.

## KEY POINTS

- Your emotional experience with fibromyalgia is valid.
- Counselling may be a great option, especially if you've experienced trauma.
- If you pursue counselling, choose a registered mental health professional (psychotherapist, psychologist, social worker, psychiatrist).
- Deficiencies in iron, vitamin B12, and vitamin D can affect mood.
- Exercising and spending time in nature have great effects on mood.

- Supplemental support for anxiety could include L-theanine, passionflower, GABA, or 5-HTP.
- Supplemental support for depression could include 5-HTP or SAMe.
- 5-HTP and SAMe have been studied specifically in fibromyalgia.
- Be sure to check with your health care provider prior to starting new supplements if you are taking any medications.

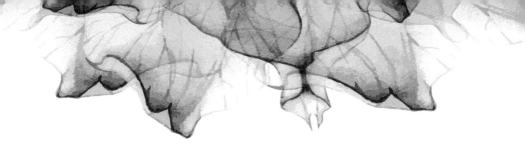

# Additional Resources

Get an electronic version of these handouts here:
https://resources.flourishingwithfibromyalgia.
com/fibromyalgia-resource-guide

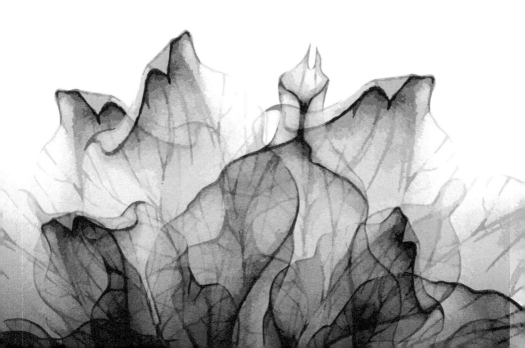

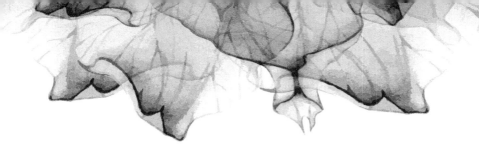

# BOOKS AND RESOURCES FOR MORE INFORMATION

## BOOK RECOMMENDATIONS

- When the Body Says No By: Gabor Maté
- Anatomy of the Spirit By: Caroline Myss
- The Fibro Manual: A Complete Fibromyalgia Treatment Guide for You and Your Doctor By: Ginerva Liptan
- The Complete Fibromyalgia Health, Diet Guide & Cookbook By: Dr. Louise McCrindle & Dr. Alison Bested
- Hope and Help for Chronic Fatigue Syndrome and Fibromyalgia By: Alison Bested, Alan Logan, and Russell Howe

## ONLINE FIBROMYALGIA RESOURCES

- National ME/FM Action Network: https://www.mefmaction.com/
- Canadian Pain Society: https://www.canadianpainsociety.ca/

- American Fibromyalgia Syndrome Association: http://www.afsafund.org/
- American Chronic Pain Association: https://www.theacpa.org/
- National Fibromyalgia & Chronic Pain Association: https://fibroandpain.org/
  - See this website for Support Groups across the U.S.
- National Fibromyalgia Partnership: http://www.fmpartnership.org/index.asp
- National Fibromyalgia Association: http://www.fmaware.org/
- European Network of Fibromyalgia Associations: https://www.enfa-europe.eu/
- Fibromyalgia Action UK: http://www.fmauk.org/
- Fibromyalgia Exercise Video: https://www.nhs.uk/conditions/nhs-fitness-studio/ms-and-fibromyalgia-pilates-exercise-video/
- Yoga Videos (Yoga with Adriene): https://www.youtube.com/user/yogawithadriene
- Widespread Pain Index and Symptom Severity Score (WPI-SSS): https://neuro.memorialhermann.org/uploadedFiles/_Library_Files/MNII/NewFibroCriteriaSurvey.pdf
- Revised Fibromyalgia Impact Questionnaire (FIQR): https://fiqrinfo.ipage.com/FIQR%20FORM.pdf
- Support Groups on Facebook
  - Fibromyalgia Canada
  - Fibromyalgia Warriors
  - Living with Fibromyalgia & Chronic Illness

## RESOURCES DISCUSSED THROUGHOUT THE BOOK

- Medication Interaction Checker: https://mytavin.com/
- Environmental Mould Investigation: https://immunolytics.com/
- Environmental Working Group Guides

- ◆ Produce (Dirty Dozen/Clean 15): https://www.ewg.org/foodnews/
- ◆ Water Filter Guide: https://www.ewg.org/tapwater/water-filter-guide.php
- ◆ Tap Water Database (U.S.): https://www.ewg.org/tapwater/
- ◆ Beauty Products: https://www.ewg.org/skindeep
- ◆ Cleaning Products: https://www.ewg.org/guides/cleaners
- ◆ Healthy Home Guide: https://www.ewg.org/healthyhomeguide/
- Environmental Working Group Healthy Living App: https://www.ewg.org/apps/
- Government of Canada Water Quality Information: https://www.canada.ca/en/health-canada/services/environmental-workplace-health/reports-publications/water-quality.html

# DOSING OF NEW SUPPLEMENTS IN FIBROMYALGIA

The motto for dosing of new treatments in fibromyalgia is: *Start Low and Go Slow*. This applies to the natural supplements discussed in this book, as well as new medications. You know your body best and you will likely have a good idea of how sensitive you are to new supplements, so you can tailor this to fit your body as you need to. As mentioned previously, liquid or powder supplement forms provide the most flexibility in dosing. Capsules can be opened and tablets can be cut, if necessary. You may also take a supplement on alternating days if you find that works better for you.

As a general rule, start with a ¼ of the target dose for two weeks. For example, if your target dose is two capsules twice per day, start with one capsule once per day.

If you are tolerating the new supplement well after the two-week trial period, increase the dose by that same amount. If we use the example of a target dose of two capsules twice per day, increase the dose to one capsule twice per day for two weeks.

If you continue to tolerate the new supplement well in the two weeks after the dose increase, you can increase the dose again following the same pattern until you reach the target dose.

If at any point you are not tolerating a dose increase, decrease the dose down to the dose you were tolerating. This is the maximum dose you should be take. When experiencing adverse effects, your body is telling you it can't handle more.

Many of my fibromyalgia patients struggle with the concept of taking a supplement, but not being able to reach the recommended dose because of sensitivity. The goal is to feel good with what you are putting into your body, not to reach a specific dose. If you are noticing benefit, the supplement is doing something regardless of how far below the recommended dose you are. As a bonus, if you feel great at a lower dose than recommended, you'll be saving money and your supplements will last longer.

The doses discussed throughout this book are maximum doses. Do not exceed these doses unless instructed to do so by a health care provider. *More does not always mean better.*

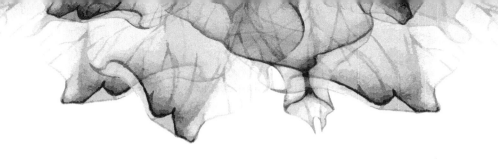

# CONDITIONS TO CONSIDER IN THE DIAGNOSIS OF FIBROMYALGIA

| | |
|---|---|
| **CONDITIONS PRESENTING WITH FATIGUE** | • Anemias<br>• Folate deficiency<br>• Vitamin B12 deficiency<br>• Iron deficiency<br>• Hepatitis<br>• HIV/AIDS<br>• Tuberculosis<br>• Epstein-Barr virus<br>• Diabetes mellitus<br>• Hypothyroidism<br>• Hyperthyroidism<br>• Addison Disease<br>• Cushing syndrome<br>• Systemic lupus erythematosus (SLE)<br>• Multiple sclerosis<br>• Myasthenia gravis<br>• Depression<br>• Hemochromatosis<br>• Sleep apnea |

| | |
|---|---|
| **CONDITIONS PRESENTING WITH PAIN** | • Polymyalgia rheumatica<br>• Ehlers-Danlos Syndrome<br>• Peripheral neuropathies<br>• Nerve entrapment syndromes<br>• TMJ syndrome<br>• Low back pain |
| **CONDITIONS PRESENTING WITH BOTH FATIGUE AND PAIN** | • Vitamin D deficiency<br>• Magnesium deficiency<br>• Lyme disease<br>• Rheumatoid arthritis<br>• Autoimmune myositis (polymyositis/ dermatomyositis)<br>• Parkinson disease<br>• Medication or substance-induced pain and fatigue<br>• Cancer<br>• Heavy metal toxicity<br>• Mould and mycotoxin illness<br>• Sjogren's syndrome<br>• Hyperparathyroidism |

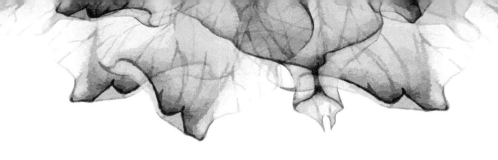

# HOW TO INCREASE IRON STORES WITH FOOD

## RECOMMENDED DIETARY ALLOWANCE IRON INTAKE (MG/DAY)[180]

| LIFE STAGE | MALES | FEMALES |
|---|---|---|
| 7 to 12 months | 11 | 11 |
| 1 to 3 years | 7 | 7 |
| 4 to 8 years | 10 | 10 |
| 9 to 13 years | 8 | 8 |
| 14 to 18 years | 11 | 15 |
| 19 to 50 years | 8 | 18 |
| 51 years and over | 8 | 8 |
| Pregnancy | N/A | 27 |
| Breastfeeding | N/A | 9 |

*Note: Correcting deficiencies requires more than the Recommended Dietary Allowance.

# FOODS SOURCES RICH IN IRON[181]

| FOOD GROUP | EXAMPLES |
|---|---|
| *HEME IRON SOURCES* | |
| Meat | Beef, pork, poultry, lamb, duck, venison |
| Organ Meat | Liver, kidney |
| Seafood | Oysters, shrimp, octopus, clams, scallops, crab, sardines |
| Fish | Mackerel, trout, bass, tuna, sardines |
| Eggs | Chicken, duck, quail |
| *NON-HEME IRON SOURCES* | |
| Legumes | Lentils (red, green, brown), black-eyed peas, split peas, chickpeas, soybeans, beans (black, white, pinto, kidney, lima) |
| Nuts and Nut Butters | Almonds, cashews, hazelnuts, pistachios, soy nuts |
| Seeds and Seed Butters | Pumpkin seeds, sunflower seeds, sesame seeds |
| Grain Products | Enriched cereals, enriched pasta, oatmeal |

| | |
|---|---|
| Soy Products | Soy milk, soy yogurt, tempeh, tofu (extra firm has more than other varieties) |
| Vegetables | Cooked spinach, asparagus, beets, beet greens, turnip greens, green peas |
| Other | Blackstrap molasses |

There are two types of iron: heme (from meat products) and non-heme (from plant sources). The body absorbs heme iron better than non-heme iron. To increase iron stores through the diet, we want to increase iron absorption and decrease malabsorption. See below for tips on how to do this.

## INCREASE IRON ABSORPTION BY:

- Eating foods containing vitamin C with iron supplements and iron-containing foods. Vitamin C helps the body absorb iron.
  - Examples of good sources of vitamin C include bell peppers, strawberries, kiwi, orange, grapefruit, lemons, tomatoes, broccoli, etc.
- Increasing protein to adequate levels for your weight and activity level. The amino acids lysine, histidine, cysteine and methionine all increase iron absorption.
- Cook using iron cookware. The acid in foods seems to pull some iron out of the cast-iron pots. Simmering acidic foods, such as tomato sauce, in an iron pot can increase the iron content of the brew over tenfold. Cooking foods containing other acids, such as vinegar, red wine, lemon or lime juice, in an iron pot can also increase the iron content of the final mixture.

## DECREASE MALABSORPTION BY:

- Avoiding tannin-containing foods/drinks when eating iron-rich foods or taking iron supplements (black tea, coffee, rhubarb). Tannins can bind to iron, making it more difficult for the body to absorb.
- Avoid consuming dairy and iron-rich foods together, as calcium competes with iron for absorption.
- Avoid or minimize oxalates (raw spinach, rhubarb, beets) and phytates (bran and whole grains), as well as carbonate (in carbonated beverages).
- Eating excess fiber and legumes with iron-rich foods will decrease absorption. Examples of foods to avoid consuming with iron-rich foods include soybeans, tofu, soy protein, split peas and lentils. If you are eating these foods with iron-rich foods, be sure to eat them with Vitamin C containing foods.
- Avoid the use of antacids, since stomach acid is required to release iron from foods.

## HINTS/TIPS:

- Add mandarin, tomato or kiwi slices to spinach salads.
- Add raisins, currents, apricots and other dried fruit to cereals and salads, and consume as a snack.
- Use beans/peas in soups.
- Limit pop consumption, especially with meals.
- Have a source of protein with each meal.

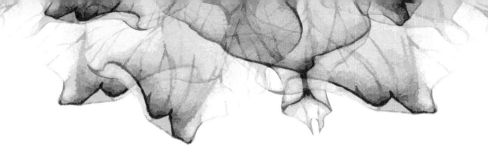

# THE LOW-FODMAP DIET

## WHAT DOES FODMAP STAND FOR?

- FODMAP stands for Fermentable Oligo-Di-Monosaccharides and Polyols.
- FODMAPs are carbohydrates (sugars) that are found in foods.
- Not all carbohydrates are considered FODMAPs.

## THE FODMAPS IN THE DIET ARE:

- Fructose found in fruits, honey, High Fructose Corn Syrup (HFCS), etc.
- Lactose found in dairy products
- Fructans found in wheat, onion, garlic, etc.
  - Fructans are also known as inulin
- Galactans found in beans, lentils, legumes such as soy, etc.

- Polyols found in sweeteners containing sorbitol, mannitol, xylitol, maltitol, stone fruits such as avocado, apricots, cherries, nectarines, peaches, plums, etc.

FODMAPs are osmotic, meaning they pull water into the intestinal tract. FODMAPs may not be digested or absorbed well and could be fermented upon by bacteria in the intestinal tract when eaten in excess.

Symptoms of gas, bloating, cramping and/or diarrhea may occur in those who could be sensitive to the effects of FODMAPs. A low-FODMAP diet may help reduce symptoms, which will limit foods high in fructose, lactose, fructans, galactans and polyols.

The low-FODMAP diet is often used in those with Irritable Bowel Syndrome (IBS). The diet also has potential use in those with similar symptoms arising from other digestive disorders such as inflammatory bowel disease.

This diet will also limit fiber as some high-fiber foods have also high amounts of FODMAPs. Fiber is a component of complex carbohydrates that the body cannot digest, found in plant-based foods such as beans, fruits, vegetables, whole grains, etc.

## LOW-FODMAP FOOD CHOICES

| FOOD GROUP | FOODS TO EAT | FOODS TO LIMIT |
|---|---|---|
| Meats and Alternatives (nuts, seeds, beans) | Chicken, turkey, fish, shellfish, canned tuna, eggs, egg whites, beef, lamb, pork, nuts, seeds, nut butters, flaxseeds | Foods made with high FODMAP fruit sauces or with HFCS, beans, black-eyed peas, hummus, lentils, pistachios |
| Dairy | Lactose free dairy, small amounts of: cream cheese, half and half, hard cheeses (cheddar, colby, parmesan, swiss), mozzarella, sherbet | Buttermilk, chocolate, cottage cheese, ice cream, creamy/ cheesy sauces, milk (from cow, sheep or goat), sweetened condensed milk, evaporated milk, soft cheeses (brie, ricotta), sour cream, whipped cream, yogurt |
| Dairy Alternatives | Almond milk, rice milk, rice milk, ice cream | Coconut milk, coconut cream, soy products |

| | | |
|---|---|---|
| Grains | Gluten-free grains and flours: Amaranth, buckwheat, rice, millet quinoa, sorghum, teff, gluten-free oats; and products made from these grains (breads, hot/cold cereals, crackers, noodles, pastas, quinoa, pancakes, tortillas), rice, tapioca | Chicory root, inulin, grains with HFCS or Gluten containing grains (wheat, spelt, kamut, barley, rye, triticale, oats), wheat flours (terms for wheat flour: bromated, durum, enriched, farina, graham, semolina, white flours), flour tortillas |
| Fruits | Bananas, berries, cantaloupe, grapes, grapefruit, honeydew, kiwi, kumquat, lemon, lime, mandarin, orange, passion fruit, pineapple, rhubarb, tangerine | Avocado, apples, applesauce, apricots, dates, canned fruit, cherries, dried fruits, figs, guava, lychee, mango, nectarines, pears, papaya, peaches, plums, prunes, persimmon, watermelon |
| Vegetables | Bamboo shoots, bell peppers, bok choy, cucumbers, carrots, celery, corn, eggplant, lettuce, leafy greens, pumpkin, potatoes, squash, yams, (butternut, winter), tomatoes, zucchini | Artichokes, asparagus, beets, leeks, broccoli, Brussels sprouts, cabbage, cauliflower, fennel, green beans, mushrooms, okra, snow peas, summer squash |

| | | |
|---|---|---|
| Beverages | Water, coffee, tea, low FODMAP fruit/ vegetable juices (limit to 1/2 cup at a time) | Any with HFCS, high FODMAP fruit/ vegetable juices, fortified wines (sherry, port) |
| Seasonings, Condiments | Most spices and herbs, homemade broth, butter, chives, olive oil, white vinegar, balsamic vinegar, garlic flavored oil, olives, mayonnaise, pepper, salt, sugar, maple syrup without HFCS, mustard, low FODMAP salad dressings, soy sauce, marinara sauce (small amounts) | HFCS, agave, chutneys, coconut, garlic, honey, jams, jellies, molasses, onions, pickle, relish, high FODMAP fruit/ vegetable sauces, salad dressings made with high FODMAPs, artificial sweeteners: sorbitol, mannitol, isomalt, xylitol (cough drops, gums, mints) |
| Desserts | Any made with allowed foods | Any with HFCS or made with foods to limit |

## TIPS FOR A LOW-FODMAP DIET:

- Follow the diet for 6 weeks. After this, add high FODMAP foods individually back into the diet in small amounts to identify foods that could be *triggers* to your symptoms. Limit foods that trigger your symptoms.
  - See the Food Reintroduction section of the Elimination Diet handout for more details.

- Read food labels. Avoid foods made with high FODMAPs such as high FODMAP fruits, HFCS, honey, inulin, wheat, soy, etc. However, a food could be an overall low FODMAP food if a high FODMAP food listed as the last ingredient.
- Buy gluten-free grains. However, you do not need to follow a completely gluten-free diet, as the focus is on FODMAPs, not gluten. Look for gluten-free grains made with low FODMAPs, such as Amaranth, buckwheat, rice, millet quinoa, sorghum, teff, gluten-free oats. Avoid gluten-free grains made with high FODMAPs.
- Limit serving sizes for high FODMAP fruits/vegetables and high fiber/low FODMAP foods such as quinoa, if you have symptoms after eating these foods. The symptoms could be related to eating large amounts of low FODMAPs or fiber all at once.

## LOW-FODMAP MEALS AND SNACK IDEAS

- Gluten-free waffle with walnuts, blueberries, and maple syrup without HFCS
- Eggs scrambled with spinach, bell peppers, and cheddar cheese
- Oatmeal topped with sliced banana, berries, almonds, and brown sugar
- Fruit smoothie blended with lactose-free yogurt and strawberries
- Rice pasta with chicken, tomatoes, and spinach topped with pesto sauce
- Chicken salad made with chicken, lettuce, bell peppers, cucumbers, tomatoes, and balsamic vinegar salad dressing
- Turkey wrap with gluten-free tortilla, sliced turkey, lettuce, tomato, a slice of cheddar cheese, mayonnaise, or mustard

- Ham and Swiss cheese sandwich on gluten-free bread, with mayonnaise or mustard
- Quesadilla with corn or gluten-free tortilla and cheddar cheese
- Beef and vegetable stew, made with homemade broth, beef, allowed vegetables

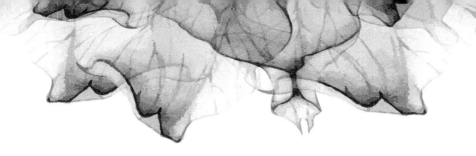

# HOW TO PRACTICE SLEEP HYGIENE

## GETTING READY FOR BED

- Make your room as dark as possible.
    - You shouldn't be able to see your hand in front of your face.
    - If you use an alarm clock, turn it away from you. Why? When light hits your skin, it disrupts circadian rhythm of the pineal gland. The pineal gland is a gland within the brain that releases melatonin, your sleep hormone. The response of the brain to light hinders the production of melatonin.
- Use low lighting in your bedroom.
    - Avoid using overhead lights and lamps with high-wattage bulbs.
- Be aware of electromagnetic fields (EMFs) in your bedroom.

- ◆ Electromagnetic fields disrupt the pineal gland, specifically the production of melatonin and serotonin. Digital alarm clocks and other electrical devices emit EMFs. If you use them, leave them at least three feet away from your bed.
- Turn off the TV.
- Use your bed for sleeping and intimacy only.
- Create bedroom *Zen*.
  - ◆ Try removing clutter, homework, calendars, etc.
  - ◆ If you can, think about painting the room in earthy tones or making it your relaxing place.
  - ◆ You can use lavender or peppermint essential oils.
- Choose comfortable, soothing bedding.
  - ◆ Nothing that makes you too warm or itchy.
- Avoid using a loud alarm clock.
  - ◆ Waking up suddenly to the blaring wail of an alarm clock can be a shock to your body. You'll also find you'll feel groggier when you rouse in the middle of a sleep cycle.
  - ◆ If you get enough sleep regularly, an alarm clock will not be necessary.
  - ◆ If you do use an alarm, you should wake just before it goes off.
  - ◆ You can use a sunrise alarm, an alarm that gradually gets louder, or an alarm that plays soothing classical music. A sunrise alarm is an alarm clock with a natural light built in that simulates a sunrise.
- If you go to the bathroom during the night, keep the lights off.
  - ◆ Brief exposure to light can shut down the melatonin production.
  - ◆ If you really need a light, use a dim nightlight and keep this outside of the bedroom.

- Think about getting a comfortable mattress and pillow.
  - Consider how long you've had your mattress and pillow.
  - Mattresses should typically be replaced at least every 7–10 years.
  - The lifetime of pillows depends on what material they are made from, but should be replaced every six months to two years, depending on the quality of your pillow. If you are experiencing neck pain or are physically uncomfortable while sleeping, it may be time to invest in a new pillow.

## NOW THAT YOUR ROOM IS READY, LET'S TALK ABOUT SLEEP!

- Establish regular sleeping hours.
  - Try to get up each morning and go to bed every night at roughly the same time. Over sleeping can be as bad as sleep deprivation, how you feel each day indicates of how much sleep is right for you.
- Sleep nude (or as close to it as possible).
  - Wearing tight clothing (bras, underwear, girdles) will increase your body temperature and interfere with melatonin release while you sleep.
  - You can also try a loose t-shirt and shorts or a nightgown.
- Get to bed by 11:00 p.m.
  - Stress glands (the adrenals) recharge or recover between 11:00 p.m. and 1:00 a.m., so going to bed before 11:00 p.m. is optimal for rebuilding your adrenal reserves.
  - If it takes you some time to fall asleep, aim to be in bed around 10:00 p.m. to account for the time it takes you to fall asleep.

- ◆ Start by going to bed 15–30 minutes earlier each night until you reach this goal.
- Sleep 8–10 hours a night.
  - ◆ Some people just need more sleep than others. If you can wake with an alarm and feel rested, you're probably getting the right amount of sleep for you.
  - ◆ With fibromyalgia, you often need more sleep than people without fibromyalgia.
- See the light first thing in the morning.
  - ◆ Daylight and morning sounds are key signals that help waken your brain.
  - ◆ Opening the blinds is the proper way to reset your body clock and ensure that your melatonin levels drop back to *awake mode* until the evening. Also, the exposure to morning light is one of the easiest ways to get a boost of energy.
- Keep household lighting dim from dinnertime until you go to sleep.
  - ◆ This simple step not only prepares your body and hormones for sleep, but it also helps your digestion, as it puts your body into *rest and digest mode.*

## NOW YOU'RE SLEEPING, BUT IF YOU'RE HAVING TROUBLE STAYING ASLEEP

- Avoid stimulating activities before bed, such as watching TV, using the computer, or using your cell phone.
  - ◆ Computer and cell phone use in the evening raises dopamine and noradrenalin, which stimulate the brain. In the evening you need to engage in activities that

make you more serotonin dominant, such as reading or meditation.

- ◆ Choose relaxing reading materials that have nothing to do with work!
- ◆ Avoid listening to the news in the evening.
- ◆ Stop all your work-related activities at least two hours before bed.

- Develop a calming bedtime routine.
  - ◆ Breaking bad habits often requires making good ones. Reading something spiritual or listening to soft music can become cues for your mind to relax.
  - ◆ Choose nighttime reading carefully. Make sure it isn't emotionally-charged material, unless it makes you feel good and helps take your mind off stress.

- If you cannot sleep and are feeling frustrated, get out of bed and do something else
  - ◆ We want to avoid your brain associating bedtime with frustration, as this can prevent progress to restful sleep.
  - ◆ Staring at the clock will also make you feel worse, so turn it around.
  - ◆ Try getting up for a while and reading or meditating. Keep the lights low and screens off, to prevent disruptions to melatonin production.
  - ◆ With fibromyalgia, rest is very important, even if you can't sleep. If you're lying awake in bed, but not feeling frustrated, remind yourself that you are still helping your body by resting.

- Make a to-do list or try writing in a journal before bed.
  - ◆ If you have problems sleeping because you feel that you have one million things to do, then write everything down! Emptying those thoughts onto paper may help to clear your mind. You can keep your lists and writings

or you can throw them away, whichever you find the most calming.

- Exercise at the right time.
    - Exercising within three hours of bedtime may be too stimulating and can impede your ability to fall asleep.
    - Yoga is an exception to this rule, because it is less stimulating than cardiovascular exercise.
    - Working out 3–6 hours before bed can help maximize the benefits of exercise on sleep, since the body increases deep sleep to compensate for the physical stress of your workout.
    - Exercise also promotes healthy sleep patterns, because of its positive effect on body temperature. After a workout, our body gradually cools down, which naturally makes us feel sleepy.
    - To relax muscles and trigger the sleep response after exercise, try a hot bath with Epsom salts. Soak in comfortably hot water with 1–2 cups of Epsom salts for at least 20 minutes.
- Exercise your mind too.
    - Try Sudoku puzzle or a daily crossword.
    - People who are mentally stimulated during the day feel a need to sleep to maintain their performance.
- Take a hot bath or shower before bed.
    - Your body will naturally cool down after a hot bath or shower, making you feel sleepier.
    - Take a hot bath/shower about two hours before bedtime, keeping the water hot for at least 25 minutes.
    - You can also add Epsom salts to a bath to detox the body and relax your muscles.
- Rest periodically throughout the day.

- ◆ If you are over-doing it throughout the day, you will feel wired once it's time for bed. This is because your fight-or-flight response has kicked in and your body thinks it needs to be on alert for impending danger.
- ◆ Remember in fibromyalgia, the stress response is abnormal and we're trying to re-train the body to respond appropriately.
- ◆ Schedule your rest periods through the day and be sure you are resting when you need to. This will help to ensure you are sleeping well at night.
- Avoid caffeine.
  - ◆ Caffeine is metabolized at different rates in different people.
  - ◆ A dose of caffeine usually takes 15 to 30 minutes to take effect and lasts for 4–5 hours. In some people it may last much longer, making consumption of caffeine in the afternoon a bad idea.
  - ◆ If you must have it, have it in the morning.
  - ◆ Caffeine may also negatively affect the natural release cycle of cortisol, which is generally highest in the morning and lowest in the evening.
  - ◆ Cortisol release rises slightly at 2am and 4am, and then hits its peak around 6am. If this pattern is disrupted, you may awaken at these times and find you are unable to fall back asleep.
- Avoid bedtime snacks high in sugar or simple carbohydrates.
  - ◆ Breads, cereals, muffins, cookies, or other baked goods prompt short-term spike in blood sugar, followed by a sugar crash later on.
  - ◆ A drop in blood sugar drop causes the release of adrenalin, cortisol, and growth hormone to regulate

blood glucose levels. These stimulate the brain, making you become more awake.

- ◆ Try to avoid eating for at least two hours before going to bed. If you need to eat, choose a snack containing protein, such as an apple with nut butter.
- ◆ Tryptophan is widespread within protein sources and is converted to serotonin and melatonin, which will help you feel sleepy. Natural sugars from the fruit may help the tryptophan reach your brain and take effect more readily. Having a snack containing protein will also help to stabilize your blood sugars through the night and prevent you from awaking because of a blood sugar drop.

- Try to avoid fluids within two hours of bedtime.
  - ◆ Avoiding the drinks may help you avoid waking to go to the washroom at night.
- Go easy on the alcohol.
  - ◆ The body metabolizes alcohol as you sleep, which can cause sleep interruption.
  - ◆ Alcohol appears to affect brain chemicals that influence sleep, shortens total sleep time, and prevents you from failing into deeper stages of sleep (where you do most of your healing).
  - ◆ One ounce or more within two hours of bedtime may disrupt sleep.
- Complete your meditation or visualizations in the evening.
  - ◆ Helps to calm the mind, relax your muscles, and allow restful sleep to ensue.

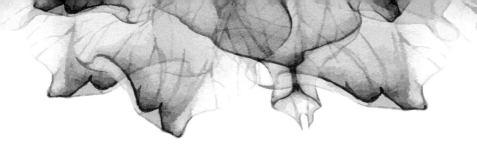

# HOW TO INCREASE YOUR PROTEIN INTAKE

Protein is essential to the body for repair, to enable the immune system to function, and for recovery from illness. Good vegetarian sources of protein include: cereals, nuts and seeds, soy products (soy milk, tofu, tempeh, etc.) and pulses (edible seeds in the legume family). Milk, yogurt, cheese, and free-range eggs are also excellent non-vegan protein sources.

## TIPS FOR EATING PROTEIN:

- Ensure that you include a protein source at each meal.
- Eat a variety of protein sources to ensure you get all the essential amino acids.

## PROTEIN SOURCES

- Include *dried beans and peas* at least three to four times a week. Choose options such as lentils, chickpeas, split peas, navy beans, adzuki beans, split mung beans, white beans, kidney beans, black beans, etc. Tahini (ground sesame seeds) and hummus (ground chickpeas) are excellent with vegetables as a snack. If you have difficulty digesting beans and lentils, try cooking and mashing them.
- *Raw nuts and seeds* are a source of protein, healthy fats, and minerals.
- Try *nut butters.* There are many more available other than peanut butter. Try others, such as hazelnut, almond, or cashew nut butter.
- *Non-farmed, cold-water ocean fish,* especially herring, sardines, wild caught salmon, and rainbow trout.
- *Grass-fed (hormone-free and antibiotic-free) meats* such as chicken, turkey, lamb, beef, veal, wild game, etc.
- *Organic soy products* are excellent and easily digested sources of protein. Tofu, miso, tempeh, wheat-free tamari soy sauce. Choose organic and non-GMO sources wherever possible.
- *Organic free-range eggs.* Do not overcook eggs or consume raw eggs. You get the most benefit from eggs if you consume both the yolk and the egg whites.
- *Dairy products,* if well tolerated, can provide additional protein. Greek yogurt and Skyr yogurt are higher in protein compared to regular yogurt. Choose unsweetened varieties and add in fruit for flavour. Cheese also provides protein, but is higher in saturated fats and should be limited.
- *Grain Products,* such as amaranth and quinoa, are great plant sources of protein.

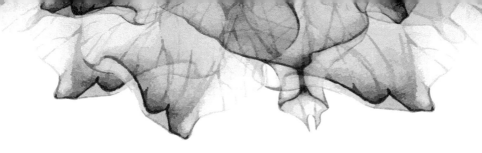

# ENERGY CONSERVATION: HOW TO PACE YOUR ACTIVITIES

Pacing involves working within the limits of the energy you have that day and finding ways to save energy where you can. Dr. Bested developed a tool called the Activity Log and Functional Capacity Scale that is used to track energy levels, activities throughout the day, and ability to function. It can be accessed on the internet via: http://mecfsassist.weebly.com/activity-log--functional-capacity-scale.html. This is the tool we will use when practicing pacing.

## Step 1: Record Your Hours of Sleep and Sleep Quality.

Under the day you are starting your activity log, record the number of hours you slept and the quality of your sleep on a scale of 1 to 5, with 1 being very poor and 5 being very good sleep.

## Step 2: Rate Your Energy at the Beginning of the Day.

At the start of your day, rate your energy on a scale of 0 to 10, based on where you fit on the functional capacity scale included with the activity log.[80] Record this before you do anything else.

## Step 3: Adjust the Times on the Left-Hand Side to Fit Your Schedule.

If you normally wake around 10a.m., adjust the times on the side accordingly, starting with 10a.m. Each time slot represents an hour of your day.

## Step 4: Record Your Activities and Functional Capacity Scale Rating throughout the Day.

The first few times you fill out the activity log, you may want to record your activities as you go and see how your functional capacity scale rating changes throughout the day. Later on, you can use the activity log to schedule your day and ensure you aren't pushing yourself beyond your limits. Every hour, record your activity and what your functional capacity scale rating is at that time. For example, in the 12p.m. slot you may write:

Ate lunch – 20 mins
Rest – 20 mins
Cleaned up – 20 mins
Functional Capacity Scale Rating = 3

You can develop your own short form to make filling out the activity log faster (for example, write "R" for rest and "C" for cleaning). I highly recommend recording your activities and functional capacity ratings as you go. If you try to record it all at the end of the day, you will not be able to remember how you were feeling in the moment.

## Step 5: Record the Number of Minutes You Exercised and the Number of Useable Hours in the Day.

Record the number of minutes you walked or exercised and the number of usable hours in the day. The useable hours in a day are hours when you are not asleep or resting with eyes closed.[80] While these numbers can be difficult to see at first, they are your starting point. It will be encouraging when you see these numbers go up and know you're on the right path.

## Step 6: Record Your Functional Capacity Scale Rating at the End of the Day.

Just before going to bed, record how you're feeling based on the functional capacity scale. Over time, we want to work on keeping your functional capacity rating consistent and prevent it from decreasing throughout the day.

## Step 7: Use Your Activity Log Daily.

Over time, you will be able to see patterns of when you pushed yourself too far and ended up with lower functional capacity ratings for the following days. You can start to identify where your limits are and how to work with them. You may even be able to identify which tasks are too much for you and work on strategies around them, either by asking for help with those tasks or by breaking them up into smaller chunks. You'll begin to see how important sleep is and how much it affects your ability to function the next day.

To help with identifying crashes and limits, it can be useful to colour-code your activity logs. For example, colouring low-energy times with red (rated as 0 to 3 on the functional capacity scale), moderate-energy times with yellow (rated as 4 to 7 on the scale), and high-energy times with green (rated as 8 to 10 on the scale) may provide a striking visual of how you're doing and where you can improve.

## Step 8: Use Your Activity Log to Schedule Your Day.

After completing a few activity logs, it's likely that you will be able to identify where you're overexerting yourself and ending up with lower functional capacity ratings at the end of the day. Ideally, we want you to start and end the day with around the same functional capacity rating. I know that sounds crazy, since what you really want is to be improving. The improvements will come over time, but to start with we want to conserve the energy you have. This concept is similar to saving your allowance, rather than blowing it all as soon as you get it. Over time, you will notice an upward trend in your functional capacity ratings if you're working within your limits during the day and implementing the other strategies in this book.

Using the activity logs you've already completed, you'll want to try to balance your day based on your functional capacity ratings. Some people find they can do more in the morning and then need to rest more in the afternoon and evening, or vice versa. If you function better in the morning, schedule your more challenging tasks in the morning and less energy-intensive tasks in the afternoon. Make sure you are scheduling rest periods throughout the day to recover from the tasks you are performing and maintain your functional capacity rating. Rest means that you are lying down with your eyes closed or sleeping. Activities such as watching TV or reading are low-energy activities, not rest. Rest periods don't necessarily have to be long but may need to be frequent. Find what works for you so that you can maintain the energy gains you will achieve.

## Warning about Activity Logs

Activity logs can be emotionally triggering at first. It can be very difficult to see how little you're accomplishing in a day. I encourage you to stick with it. As you make improvements, compare your activity logs from when you began, or when you were in a crash, to how you feel when you are doing well. This will be proof that when you take care of yourself, you can make improvements in your health, and will provide encouragement to keep working on it.

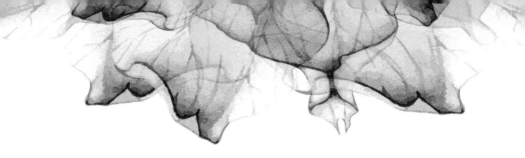

# ENERGY CONSERVING TIPS AND TRICKS

## GENERAL

- Break big jobs into smaller chunks to make them more manageable.
    - For example:
        - Day 1: Sort laundry
        - Day 2: Wash and dry
        - Day 3: Fold and put away
- Take frequent breaks and take breaks before you feel tired.
- Nap as needed throughout the day.
- Learn to say no and set boundaries.
- Opt for short outings and social events where possible.
- Plan rest days after big events.
- Use an activity tracking watch (such as a FitBit) to help with pacing.
- Never walk with empty hands.

> ◆ If you are getting up, bring something with you that needs to be put away or thrown out.

## PERSONAL HYGIENE

- Use an electric toothbrush, instead of a manual one for a deeper clean and less arm muscle exertion.
- Sit in the bath or use a shower chair instead of standing in shower.

## HOUSE KEEPING

- Hire a housekeeper, if possible.
- Avoid completing marathon cleaning or chore sessions.
- Assign chores to family members.
- Get your kids involved, as it's important they learn these skills too.
- Invest in a robot vacuum.
- Place disinfectant wipes in all bathrooms for quick cleans.

## COOKING AND MEAL PREP

- Utilize a healthy food delivery or meal service.
- Place grocery orders online and pick them up (or have a family member pick them up) to prevent long shopping excursions.
- Order dry goods and household items online and have them shipped to you.
- Snack often instead of preparing big meals when not feeling well.
- When you are cooking a meal, cook extra and freeze it for later.
- If you are planning to cook a meal, prepare it during the time of day you have more energy.

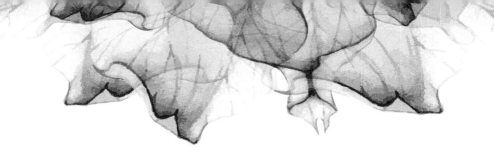

# HEALTHY MINDSET EXERCISES

## ONE DAY VISUALIZATION

The purpose of this exercise is to visualize what your life would look like if you'd never been diagnosed with fibromyalgia. The goal is not to discourage you, although I know it can feel that way when you're thinking of all of the things you can't do now. It's to give you points of reference for when you're on your journey to health. These are what you're working towards and they will be your points of celebration once you get there. There will be many small points of celebration, but these will be your big ones. These are the ones that will keep you going when it's beginning to feel like too much work. Pull out your *One Day Visualization* and remind yourself how much you deserve that life.

**Step 1: Create Your One Day Visualization**

Consider the questions below and put this life into pictures or words (whichever you prefer). This exercise is not designed to discourage you, but to give you goals to work towards when your health journey feels like it isn't going well and you feel like giving up. Once you have your *One Day Visualization*, we will break it into smaller chunks to work towards.

*Questions to Consider:*

- What your life would look like if you'd never been diagnosed with fibromyalgia, better yet if you'd never heard of it?
- What would you have accomplished?
- What would you have done differently?
- Who would you be spending your free time with?
- Are there any activities or hobbies that you gave up that you wish you continued?
- Would you be working? If so, what would you be doing?
- Would you have a family?
- Would you travel? Where to?

**Step 2: Identify a Small Part of Your One Day Visualization that You Want to Work Towards Within the Next Six Months.**

Next, I want you to identify a small part of your *one day visualization* that you want to work towards within the next six months. Recovery looks different for everyone, so timelines are flexible. Say, for example, you want to be able to go to the movie theatre and enjoy a whole film without crashing the next day or coming home feeling awful. That will be your six-month goal. Every time you're working on something for your health, whether it is taking your supplements, eating a stricter diet than you're used to, or pacing your activities and it's feeling like too much, remember your six-month goal. Baby steps will get you there, and it will feel so good when you've reached your short-term goal.

## Step 3: Periodically Revisit Your One Day Visualization.

Revisit your One Day Visualization periodically to check in on your progress. Are you getting closer to your goal? If not, is there something in your health plan that you need to change? Once you achieve your six-month goal, celebrate! Then set a new six-month goal and begin working towards it.

## POSITIVE AFFIRMATIONS

Negative self-talk is very common and can be incredibly emotionally draining. It can rob you of any motivation you once had to get better when that little voice inside your head keeps telling you that "you can't do it", "it's too hard", and "you're not worth it". Whether you've internalized this self-talk from abuse in your past or whether you're unsure where it came from, it's not serving you and it's time to get rid of it.

Positive affirmations are a great way to drown out that negative voice. The more often you combat that negative voice with positive alternatives, the more likely you are to believe the positive thoughts. Doing positive affirmations and engaging in self-love can feel unnatural at first. If this is the case for you, I recommend framing your positive affirmations into phrases you would tell someone dear to you, whether it's your best friend, your child, or your significant other. A common positive affirmation I hear people use often is "I am enough". While you are definitely enough, I wouldn't tell my best friend that she is enough. That just doesn't sound good enough for her. I would tell her something like "You deserve everything you've ever wanted in life and more" or "You deserve to be loved unconditionally and treated like a queen". Find a phrase that works for you and use that. Say it out loud, repeat it in your head, put it on your mirror, and read it before you go to bed. Consistency is key with a positive affirmation practice.

If that first method still feels like too much for you, a simple reminder to your body and your mind of "I am safe" can bring a state of calm. Remember how we discussed the abnormal stress response in fibromyalgia and how we need to train your body to respond properly to stress? Your body forgets that it is, in this moment, safe. You may need to remind it when you're feeling stressed or anxious. Although you have worries and stresses, you are not in immediate danger, and you are safe.

## MEDITATIONS AND DEEP BREATHING

Meditations and deep breathing are an important exercise in calming that overactive stress response. Many people dislike meditating and find it difficult. There's a reason it's difficult. You're stuck in a stress response, and your body has forgotten how to relax. The more you practice getting your body into a more relaxed state, the more often your body will default there and the easier it will be to calm down when you're feeling stressed.

The other reason many people find meditating difficult and don't bother with it is because when we think about meditating, we picture a Buddhist monk who sits for hours in silence and meditates. At least that's what I used to picture. We do not need to meditate for hours. We don't even need to prevent our minds from wandering fully while we meditate to get benefit from it.

When I recommend meditation to my patients, I recommend they start with just two minutes per day. Most people fit this in before bedtime or first thing in the morning. Regardless of when you fit it in, you have two minutes per day to spare. What you're doing in this two-minute time frame is mostly up to you, as long as you find the practice relaxing and you're engaging in it fully. You can do deep breathing, listen to a guided meditation, or pray. A guided meditation doesn't have to be a recording telling you when to breathe. It could be a visualization of a walk through the forest or along a beach. Find a meditation that works for you and use that. My favourite apps for guided meditations are Calm and Insight Timer. Both of which are free and can be downloaded on your phone. Calm is also available as a website.

## Box Breathing

When you're practicing box breathing, you are performing actions in time segments of four seconds. Pictorial representations of this type of meditation practice show this as a box.

Step 1: Breathe in over four seconds.

Step 2: Hold your breath for four seconds.

Step 3: Exhale your breath over four seconds.

Step 4: Hold for four seconds.

Step 5: Repeat as many times as you wish.

## Belly Breathing

Belly breathing is a form of deep breathing that involves taking a breath deep enough to expand the stomach. This gets fresh oxygen into the lower portions of your lungs, where air can stagnate. Inhaling this deeply takes most people at least five seconds. Some people place their hand on their abdomen to feel it expanding. Once you have inhaled as deeply as you can, hold your breath for three seconds, and then exhale slowly. Repeat this practice as many times as you wish.

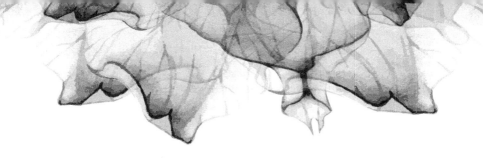

# THE ELIMINATION DIET

The elimination diet should be followed for a minimum of three weeks. Most will obtain clearer results if the elimination diet is followed for six weeks, before strategically re-introducing foods.

## FOOD GUIDELINES

- Choose organic fruits and vegetables if possible.
- Make sure you wash produce thoroughly to remove pesticide residues and contaminants, using cold water and a scrubbing brush (only for firm produce items).
- Be sure to read labels thoroughly to find added ingredients and avoid anything with sugar, glucose, fructose, EDTA, flavouring, colour, or any other preservatives.
- Identify foods you eat on the *Foods to Avoid* list and switch these out for *Foods to Eat* to make the elimination diet easier.

## Vegetables

| FOODS TO EAT | FOODS TO AVOID |
|---|---|
| • Beets, leeks, Brussels sprouts, green beans, turnips, bok choy, asparagus, fiddle heads, kohlrabi, okra, parsnip, peas, radish, rutabaga, squash<br>• Arugula, turnip greens, spinach, kale, collard greens, dandelion greens, romaine lettuce, radicchio, watercress<br>• Sweet potatoes and yams<br>• Try to incorporate sprouts, especially mung beans, alfalfa, and red clover, as they help with detoxification | • Tomatoes, peppers, eggplants<br>• Corn, potatoes, carrot, celery, zucchini, cauliflower, cucumber, cabbage (red and green), broccoli, swiss chard, rapini<br>• Onions, garlic, mushrooms<br>• Frozen, canned, or jarred vegetables<br><br>**Note:** If ragweed allergy is present, eliminate artichokes, iceberg lettuce, sunflower seeds and oil, safflower oil, dandelion, chamomile, and chicory. |

Note: Can be eaten raw, steamed or baked, no frying.

## Fruits

| FOODS TO EAT | FOODS TO AVOID |
|---|---|
| • Lemon, lime, dates, avocado, figs, kiwi, kumquat, lychee, mango, nectarine, olives, papaya, passionfruit, persimmon, dragonfruit, pomegranate, prickly pear, rhubarb<br>• Blueberries, blackberries, raspberries, mulberries, cranberries<br>• Fruit sauces with no sugar added | • Citrus (oranges, grapefruit), apple, peach, plum, pear, cherry, apricot, banana, grapes, pineapple<br>• Cantaloupe, honeydew melon, watermelon<br>• Strawberries<br>• Dried fruits |

Eat fruit by itself: ½ hour before or 2 hours after a meal, unless using in fruit smoothie.

## Grains

| FOODS TO EAT | FOODS TO AVOID |
|---|---|
| • Brown rice, millet, buckwheat, quinoa, tapioca, teff, amaranth, oats, sorghum<br>• You can also eat cereals made from these grains.<br>• Brown rice pasta, quinoa pasta, buckwheat pasta<br>• Gluten Free Brands: Aiden's, Little Northern Bakehouse, Little Steam Bakery, Udi's | • All gluten-containing grains (wheat, spelt, rye, kamut, barley, couscous, pumpernickel) commonly found in breads, pasta & other products from refined flour<br>• By avoiding these foods for a few weeks, it gives your body a chance to relax. You may not even know you have an allergy to these foods because the symptoms may be so subtle. |

## Legumes

| FOODS TO EAT | FOODS TO AVOID |
|---|---|
| • All legumes (adzuki beans, navy, black, etc.)<br>• All peas (fresh, split, snap)<br>• Lentils (any variety) | • Soy beans & soy products (tofu, soy milk, soy, miso, tempeh, Textured Vegetable Protein)<br><br>**Note:** Soy is another common allergen. |

## Nuts & Seeds

| FOODS TO EAT | FOODS TO AVOID |
|---|---|
| • Brazil nuts, pecans, pine nuts, macadamia nuts, almonds<br>• Pumpkin, sesame, flax, sunflower, chia, and hemp seeds | • Peanuts, pistachios, cashews, hazelnuts, walnuts<br>• Any nuts or seeds that are salted or have added flavouring |

## Animal Products

| FOODS TO EAT | FOODS TO AVOID |
|---|---|
| • Free-range chicken & turkey (can be grain-fed, if organic not available)<br>• Organic lamb or New Zealand lamb, wild game<br>• Wild deep-water fish (salmon, halibut, cod, mackerel, sardines), whitefish, tilapia, trout | • Red meats (beef, pork, bacon), sandwich meats, hotdogs, sausage, canned meats, smoked meats, shellfish, catfish<br>• Dairy (milk, cream, sour cream, cheese, butter, yogurt)<br>• Eggs |

## Condiments

| FOODS TO EAT | FOODS TO AVOID |
|---|---|
| • Oils for cooking: grapeseed oil, coconut oil, or avocado oil<br>• On salads or steamed veggies: olive oil or flaxseed oil<br>• Herbs: basil, oregano, thyme, rosemary, bay leaves, cilantro, dill, marjoram, lemongrass<br>• Spices: cayenne, cinnamon, clove, allspice, cardamom, cumin, ginger, nutmeg, turmeric<br>• Spreads: tahini paste, apple butter, bean dips, hummus<br>• Apple cider vinegar, brown rice vinegar, fresh lemon juice (not concentrated)<br>• Sweeteners: Stevia, apple butter, natural maple syrups, honey | • Regular table salt<br>• Refined oils, margarine, shortening<br>• All sweeteners (corn syrup, brown rice syrup, molasses, brown sugar, white sugar, glucose, maltose, malto-dextrose, aspartame, etc.)<br>• MSG<br>• Mustard<br>• Herbs: parsley<br>• Spices: aniseed, black pepper, coriander, caraway, fennel, curry, paprika<br><br>**Note:**<br><br>• This includes all desserts and all processed foods high in sugars.<br>• Do not heat flaxseed or olive oil. Instead, mix into cooked grains, drizzle over salad or steamed vegetables. Add fruits to smoothies to sweeten. |

## Beverages

| FOODS TO EAT | FOODS TO AVOID |
|---|---|
| • Filtered water, at least eight glasses<br>• 100% fruit and vegetable juices (unsweetened)<br>• Herbal teas (rooibos, peppermint, chamomile, licorice, passionflower, dandelion, milk thistle, etc.)<br>• Green tea<br>• Rice milk (unsweetened)<br>• Coconut water and unsweetened coconut milk | • Caffeinated beverages (coffee, black tea, soda)<br>• Alcohol<br>• Dairy (milk, drinkable yogurt)<br>• Soy milk<br>• All fruit drinks high in refined sugars<br>• All vegetable drinks high in salt |

Try warm water with a ¼ squeezed lemon in the water, as it aids digestion and liver detoxification.

- Drink liquids ½ hour before or one hour after eating. Consuming liquids with meals will dilute the enzymes in the stomach needed to digest the food properly.

## MEAL SUGGESTIONS

### Breakfast

Breakfast may include combinations of approved grains, meats, and fruits. Below are a few ideas:

1.  Buckwheat/millet/brown rice porridge or quinoa to this you can add cinnamon and allowed berries, a few pumpkin seeds, and rice milk.
2.  In general, add fruit, nuts and spice to porridge while it's cooking. This makes fruit and nuts more digestible and adds flavor.
3.  Fruit smoothie, blend together the following:
    a. 1 cup rice milk
    b. 1 cup of fruit (berries, mango, papaya)
    c. 1 tbsp flax oil
    d. ½ tbsp tahini
    e. A few macadamia nuts
4.  Buckwheat flakes, rice flakes, rice crisps, nutty rice, cereal with rice or nut milk.

### Lunch & Dinner

Lunch and dinner may include approved organic, grain fed chicken and turkey, wild game, fish, grains, legumes, cooked or raw vegetables, soups, and salads.

## Snacks

- Brown rice crackers or brown rice cakes with hummus, tahini with vegetable topping (sprouts, cucumber, cooked beets), avocado.
- Fruits, especially those that are seasonal.
- Raw vegetables (carrot and celery sticks).
- Handful of allowed nuts or baked sweet potato.

## SYMPTOM TRACKING

Record the date and time of the introduction of the new food. If you experience any symptoms, record the nature of the symptoms, as well as the date and time the symptoms occurred. This can help you identify how long after consuming a specific food you should expect a symptomatic reaction. This time frame can be different for different foods. It is also helpful to write down how long the symptoms lasted.

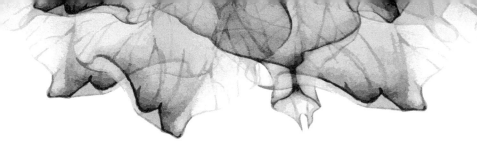

# FOOD REINTRODUCTION

Food Reintroduction occurs after the Elimination Diet has been followed for three to six weeks. Once the elimination diet ends, you will be gradually reintroducing the foods that you have been avoiding and tracking your symptoms.

Every newly introduced food or food group should be eaten during at least two of the three meals in one day for three consecutive days. If you react to the food at any point, you need to stop eating the offending food. If, however, you have no reactions after the third day you simply introduce another food group on day four.

Please note that when you react to an introduced food, you must wait until your reaction subsides before reintroducing of the next food group. Do not eat the offending food until the reintroduction of all the other food groups is over. Then challenge the offending food again at the very end.

All the foods from the Foods to Avoid category that you eliminated from your diet will be reintroduced. The order of reintroduction is up to you. I often recommend that you reintroduce your favourite foods first; however, many will recommend reintroduction of the least common allergens first.

Once you have reintroduced all the various foods into your diet, you will to go back and try eating those foods that you were sensitive to and see how you react to them. If you have any adverse reaction(s) to that food or food group, then you know that you may need to avoid that food all together or eat it sparingly.

When reintroducing foods after the elimination diet:

- Purest form of food should be introduced.
    - Example: If reintroducing dairy, reintroduce milk first, then yogurt, then cheese, etc.
- Drink adequate amounts of water (at least eight glasses per day).

How to Reintroduce Foods

- Day 1: Try to eat the new food three times/day.
- Day 2, 3, and 4: Do not eat the re-introduced food.
    - Watch for any symptoms including headaches, more pronounced fatigue, digestive issues, anxiety, irritability, sleep disturbances, mood changes, exacerbation of skin conditions, increased pain, joint pain, or other symptoms.
    - If you have a reaction, stop eating the food right away and allow symptoms to subside before reintroducing another new food. The offending food will be

reintroduced at the end of the reintroduction phase as a second challenge.

- Day 5: If you experienced no symptoms from the previously re-introduced food, re-introduce the next food.
- If the food doesn't affect you, continue consuming it, and move to the next food at the appropriate time.
- Record the following:
  - Food you re-introduced.
  - Symptoms you experienced.
  - How long after you consumed the food did the symptoms occur.
  - How long the symptoms lasted.
- Re-introduce all foods you avoided listed in the *Foods to Avoid* column.

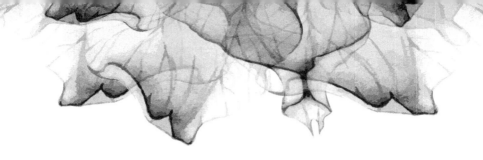

# HYDROTHERAPY FOR PAIN RELIEF AND ENERGY BOOSTS

## CONTRAST SHOWERS

### How it works:

Although we all love to have hot showers, the extended period of hot water on our body causes physiological effects. The hot water initially acts as a blood vessel dilator, meaning our blood vessels get wider, which increases blood flow. All this blood flow near the surface of our skin is why we turn red. It also increases our cellular metabolism, helping our cells get rid of toxins and waste products produced during normal activity. After five minutes of exposure to hot water, the body returns the vessel diameters to their normal measurements, but the rate of cellular metabolism stays high. Therefore, we get extra waste material being pushed into our blood, but less vessel width to push it towards the organs that filter blood. A short burst of cold water (less than a minute) also initially stimulates blood vessel dilation and cellular metabolism, but shortly after exposure to cold, both blood vessel diameter and cellular metabolism decrease.

## Benefits:

- Improves immune function.
- Increases nutrient delivery throughout the body.
- Improves circulation of blood and lymph fluid.
- Increases tissue tone.
- Helps remove toxins from the body.
- Increases energy.

## When Not to Perform:

- Do *not* do contrast showers directly after a meal.
- If you are undergoing cancer treatment.
- If you have diminished sensation.
- If you are bleeding heavily.
- If you have a vascular disease, including diabetes mellitus.

## How to do it:

- Start your shower with water as hot as you usually do, for 1 minute and 30 seconds.
- Turn the taps to water as cool as you can handle for 30 seconds.
- Change the water back to as hot as you can handle for 1 minute and 30 seconds.
- Repeat this alteration for three to five times.

- *Always* end your shower with cold water!

## How to increase its effectiveness

- It's important to start with less drastic temperature differences initially until you know how you respond to contrast showers.
- Over time, increase the difference in temperature between hot and cold to your tolerance.
- The larger the temperature difference between the hot and cold water, the greater the benefits.
- The more often you do Contrast Showers, the more benefits you will experience.

## INFRARED SAUNA

Sauna therapy can encourage detoxification, relieve pain, and improve energy levels. You must have access to a sauna for this to be an option for you. Some can access this at home or at the gym. It is ideal if you have access to a sauna with a shower nearby. If not, saunas can still be beneficial. Some people feel light-headed and dizzy during or after using a sauna. For your safety, please be sure you have someone with you the first few times you try this.

To improve your tolerance for sauna therapy, ensure you are drinking enough water throughout the session. Electrolyte water is the preferred form of hydration to replace electrolytes lost to sweating. It is generally recommended that you consume at least 1L of fluid during a sauna session.

## Cautions:

Please consult a healthcare provider prior to using a sauna if any of the following apply:

- You are pregnant or breastfeeding.
- You have surgical implants of any kind.
- You have heart disease.
- You have a seizure disorder.

Additionally, you should not use a sauna immediately after intense exercise, after alcohol or drug consumption, and within one hour of eating.

## Infrared Sauna Sessions for Pain Management

Sauna sessions can be used for pain management up to five times weekly, with most patients responding well to three sessions weekly for 30–60 minutes. If possible, start at a lower temperature to determine how you tolerate saunas. The temperature range for infrared sauna sessions is typically 43.3°C (110°F)–48.8°C (120°F). Start at a lower temperature and slowly increase the temperature over time to your tolerance.

## Instructions

1. If you are able to adjust the temperature of the sauna, set the temperature to 43.3°C (110°F) and set the timer for 60 minutes.
2. Warm the sauna up for 20 minutes prior to entering.

3. Change into a bathing suit or loose fitting, breathable clothing (i.e. shorts, tank top) and remove any metallic objects (jewellery, glasses, etc.).

4. Take a warm shower for one minute prior to entering the sauna.

5. Enter the sauna and sit for 15 minutes. You can open a ventilation window if necessary.

6. Ensure you are sipping fluids throughout your time in the sauna.

7. After 15 minutes have passed, take a cool shower for 30 seconds. Choose a temperature that feels cold, but tolerable. Similar to contrast showers, the larger the temperature difference, the bigger the effects. Be sure to start with a smaller temperature difference between hot and cold and work up to larger temperature differences.

8. Repeat steps 5–7 three more times (for a total of four cycles).

9. In the last shower of your sauna session, use soap to remove any toxins or fats released from the skin during your sauna session. Use of a loofah or scrub brush will help prevent reabsorption of anything eliminated during the sauna at this stage.

10. Rest after your sauna to ensure you are feeling well and tolerated the session well.

## Access to Infrared Sauna Without a Shower Nearby

If you have access to an infrared sauna with no shower nearby, ensure you are showering before and after your sauna session. Shorten sauna sessions to 20–30 minutes if you are not cycling between the sauna and a cool shower. Ensure you are consuming enough fluids.

## EPSOM SALT BATHS

Because of the high magnesium content, Epsom salts promote the release of lactic acid from muscle tissue. An Epsom salts bath can be helpful any time you are suffering from achiness and muscle strain. It is also an excellent idea for the evening after you have had a massage, because it helps to clear out released lactic acid.

### Muscle Tension

Muscles use oxygen and nutrients to carry out work. They also produce carbon dioxide and waste products. The principle waste product of muscle metabolism is lactic acid. Nutrients and wastes are transported to and from muscles by the blood circulation. The efficiency of this transport system is dependent upon good blood flow. Poor or insufficient blood flow causes an accumulation of lactic acid, producing tension in muscles.

### Muscle Pain

There are many types of muscle pain, but all of us are familiar with the stiff, achy feeling of a muscle that is reacting to an unusual level of exercise, a chronic strain, or build-up of stress-related tension. This achiness is caused by the development of lactic acid residues in the muscle tissue, compounded by the fact that a tight muscle clamps down on blood vessels and impedes drainage of its own tissue.

## Instructions for Taking the Bath

Epsom salts are easy to find at most pharmacies and grocery stores. Use 2–4 cups in a full bath, the temperature of which is as hot as you can comfortably tolerate. You must soak in the bath for a minimum of 20 minutes. Do not add any bathing solutions or oils and avoid using soap, as these substances will alter the chemistry of the water. After soaking for 20 minutes, you may wash off as you wish.

To replace the fluid you lose during perspiration, keep a glass of cold water beside you and sip it during the bath. If you like, you may also wring a towel in cold water and wrap it around your neck. As with any hot bath, make sure you get out of the tub slowly and carefully.

CAUTION: If you are over 50 years of age or have a diagnosed heart condition, moderate the water temperature and avoid submerging your body above heart level. Use a cold towel around your neck and keep a bucket of cold water available beside the tub for wringing. If you have any concerns about whether a hot bath will affect you adversely, please consult with your doctor before using the Epsom salts bath.

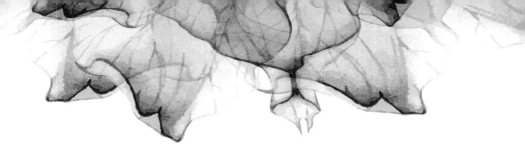

# CASTOR OIL USE INSTRUCTIONS

Castor oil has been shown to increase circulation, as well as promote elimination and healing of tissues and organs underneath the skin. It can improve digestion, immune function, and reduce swelling in injured joints and extremities. It has also been specifically used in cases of menstrual irregularities, uterine fibroid cysts, and ovarian cysts.

Note: You can either apply castor oil topically or make and apply the pack, without making the pack. Both options are equally as effective.

## CASTOR OIL TOPICAL APPLICATION

### Materials:

- Castor Oil
- White flannel or cotton cloth large enough to cover the desired area
- Heating pad, with a low setting

## Method:

- Place castor oil directly on the desired area.
- Cover the area with cotton (such as an old t-shirt for abdomen or back, a sock for the ankle, etc.).
- Rest for 20–30 minutes with a heating pad set on low, or keep the area covered and go to bed (no heating pack).

## CASTOR OIL PACK

## Materials:

- Castor Oil
- Small glass pan, with lid
- White flannel or cotton cloth large enough to cover the desired area
- Plastic, large enough to cover the flannel cloth (plastic bags are an option)
- Heating pad, with a low setting

## Method:

- Pour a small quantity of castor oil in the glass pan.
- Soak an eight inch square piece of flannel or cotton in the castor oil.
- Place the flannel on abdomen.
- Cover completely with plastic.
- Place a heating pad over plastic and set on low heat for 50–60 minutes.

- Rest while the pack is in place.
- Be careful not to fall asleep with a heating pad on.
- After removal clean the area with warm water, if desired.
- Store the pack in a covered container in the refrigerator to reuse.

## CAUTIONS

- If you experience diarrhea, decrease the amount of time with the castor oil pack on.
- If diarrhea does not subside or you develop a skin rash, discontinue use.
- Castor oil stains easily, so do not use it with nice clothing or linens.
- *Do not use on the abdomen during pregnancy or menstruation.*
- *Do not take castor oil internally.*

# REFERENCES

1.  Clauw DJ. Fibromyalgia: a clinical review. *JAMA*. 2014;311(15): 1547–1555. doi:10.1001/jama.2014.3266

2.  Fitzcharles MA, Ste-Marie PA, Pereira JX; Canadian Fibromyalgia Guidelines Committee. Fibromyalgia: evolving concepts over the past 2 decades. *CMAJ*. 2013;185(13):E645–E651. doi:10. 1503/cmaj.121414

3.  Arout CA, Sofuoglu M, Bastian LA, Rosenheck RA. Gender Differences in the Prevalence of Fibromyalgia and in Concomitant Medical and Psychiatric Disorders: A National Veterans Health Administration Study. *J Womens Health (Larchmt)*. 2018;27(8):1035–1044. doi:10.1089/jwh.2017.6622

4.  Prevalence. National Fibromyalgia Association. http://www. fmaware.org/about-fibromyalgia/prevalence/. Accessed December 9, 2019.

5.  Quick facts on fibromyalgia. American Chronic Pain Association. https://www.theacpa.org/conditions-treatments/ conditions-a-z/fibromyalgia/two-takes-on-fibro/quick-facts-on-fibromyalgia/. Accessed December 9, 2019.

6.  Bartkowska W, Samborski W, Mojs E. Cognitive functions, emotions and personality in woman with fibromyalgia. *AnthropolAnz*. 2018;75(4):271–277. doi:10.1127/anthranz/ 2018/0900

7.  Bartkowska W, Samborski W, Mojs E. Cognitive functions, emotions and personality in woman with fibromyalgia. *AnthropolAnz*. 2018;75(4):271–277. doi:10.1127/anthranz/ 2018/0900

8. Chinn S, Caldwell W, Gritsenko K. Fibromyalgia Pathogenesis and Treatment Options Update. *Curr Pain Headache Rep.* 2016;20(4):25. doi:10.1007/s11916-016-0556-x

9. Arnold LM, Fan J, Russell IJ, et al. The fibromyalgia family study: a genome-wide linkage scan study. *Arthritis Rheum.* 2013;65(4):1122–1128. doi:10.1002/art.37842

10. Park DJ, Lee SS. New insights into the genetics of fibromyalgia. *Korean J Intern Med.* 2017;32(6):984–995. doi:10.3904/kjim.2016.207

11. Park JH, Niermann KJ, Olsen N. Evidence for metabolic abnormalities in the muscles of patients with fibromyalgia. *CurrRheumatol Rep.* 2000;2(2):131–140. doi:10.1007/s11926-000-0053-3

12. Yunus MB, Kalyan-Raman UP, Kalyan-Raman K, Masi AT. Pathologic changes in muscle in primary fibromyalgia syndrome. *Am J Med.* 1986;81(3A):38–42. doi:10.1016/0002-9343(86)90872-7

13. Bengtsson A, Henriksson KG, Larsson J. Reduced high-energy phosphate levels in the painful muscles of patients with primary fibromyalgia. *Arthritis Rheum.* 1986;29(7):817–821. doi:10.1002/art.1780290701

14. Cordero MD, De Miguel M, Moreno Fernández AM, et al. Mitochondrial dysfunction and mitophagy activation in blood mononuclear cells of fibromyalgia patients: implications in the pathogenesis of the disease. *Arthritis Res Ther.* 2010;12(1):R17. doi:10.1186/ar2918

15. Cordero MD, Díaz-Parrado E, Carrión AM, et al. Is inflammation a mitochondrial dysfunction-dependent event in fibromyalgia?. *Antioxid Redox Signal.* 2013;18(7):800–807. doi:10.1089/ars.2012.4892

16. Castro-Marrero J, Cordero MD, Sáez-Francas N, et al. Could mitochondrial dysfunction be a differentiating marker between

chronic fatigue syndrome and fibromyalgia?. *Antioxid Redox Signal.* 2013;19(15):1855–1860. doi:10.1089/ars.2013.5346

17. Gerdle B, Forsgren MF, Bengtsson A, et al. Decreased muscle concentrations of ATP and PCR in the quadriceps muscle of fibromyalgia patients--a 31P-MRS study. *Eur J Pain.* 2013; 17(8):1205–1215. doi:10.1002/j.1532-2149.2013.00284.x

18. Andrés-Rodríguez L, Borràs X, Feliu-Soler A, et al. Machine Learning to Understand the Immune-Inflammatory Pathways in Fibromyalgia. *Int J Mol Sci.* 2019;20(17):4231. Published 2019 Aug 29. doi:10.3390/ijms20174231

19. Bote ME, García JJ, Hinchado MD, Ortega E. Inflammatory/ stress feedback dysregulation in women with fibromyalgia. *Neuroimmunomodulation.* 2012;19(6):343–351. doi:10.1159/ 000341664

20. Sturgill J, McGee E, Menzies V. Unique cytokine signature in the plasma of patients with fibromyalgia. *J Immunol Res.* 2014;2014:938576. doi:10.1155/2014/938576

21. Behm FG, Gavin IM, Karpenko O, et al. Unique immunologic patterns in fibromyalgia. *BMC Clin Pathol.* 2012;12:25. Published 2012 Dec 17. doi:10.1186/1472-6890-12-25

22. Martinez-Lavin M. Biology and therapy of fibromyalgia. Stress, the stress response system, and fibromyalgia. *Arthritis Res Ther.* 2007;9(4):216. doi:10.1186/ar2146

23. Pardo JV, Larson RC, Spencer RJ, et al. Exposure to Cold Unmasks Potential Biomarkers of Fibromyalgia Syndrome Reflecting Insufficient Sympathetic Responses to Stress. *Clin J Pain.* 2019;35(5):407–419. doi:10.1097/AJP.0000000000000695

24. Heim C, Ehlert U, Hellhammer DH. The potential role of hypocortisolism in the pathophysiology of stress-related bodily disorders. *Psychoneuroendocrinology.* 2000;25(1):1–35. doi:10.1016/s0306-4530(99)00035-9

25.  Rosenfeld VW, Rutledge DN, Stern JM. Polysomnography with quantitative EEG in patients with and without fibromyalgia. *J Clin Neurophysiol*. 2015;32(2):164–170. doi:10.1097/WNP. 0000000000000134

26.  Roth T, Bhadra-Brown P, Pitman VW, Roehrs TA, Resnick EM. Characteristics of Disturbed Sleep in Patients With Fibromyalgia Compared With Insomnia or With Pain-Free Volunteers. *Clin J Pain*. 2016;32(4):302–307. doi:10.1097/AJP.0000000000000261

27.  Fang SC, Wu YL, Chen SC, Teng HW, Tsai PS. Subjective sleep quality as a mediator in the relationship between pain severity and sustained attention performance in patients with fibromyalgia. *J Sleep Res*. 2019;28(6):e12843. doi:10.1111/jsr.12843

28.  Çetin B, Güleç H, Toktaş HE, Ulutaş Ö, Yılmaz SG, İsbir T. Objective measures of sleep in fibromyalgia syndrome: Relationship to clinical, psychiatric, and immunological variables. *Psychiatry Res*. 2018;263:125–129. doi:10.1016/j. psychres.2018.02.057

29.  Gracely RH, Petzke F, Wolf JM, Clauw DJ. Functional magnetic resonance imaging evidence of augmented pain processing in fibromyalgia. *Arthritis Rheum*. 2002;46(5):1333–1343. doi: 10.1002/art.10225

30.  Jensen KB, Loitoile R, Kosek E, et al. Patients with fibromyalgia display less functional connectivity in the brain's pain inhibitory network. *Mol Pain*. 2012;8:32. Published 2012 Apr 26. doi: 10.1186/1744-8069-8-32

31.  Littlejohn G, Guymer E. Neurogenic inflammation in fibromyalgia. *SeminImmunopathol*. 2018;40(3):291–300. doi: 10.1007/s00281-018-0672-2

32.  Tomasello G, Mazzola M, Bosco V, et al. Intestinal dysbiosis and hormonal neuroendocrine secretion in the fibromyalgic patient: Relationship and correlations [published online ahead of print, 2018 Sep 11]. *Biomed Pap Med Fac Univ Palacky*

*Olomouc Czech Repub.* 2018;10.5507/bp.2018.051. doi:10.5507/bp.2018.051

33. Minerbi A, Gonzalez E, Brereton NJB, et al. Altered microbiome composition in individuals with fibromyalgia. *Pain.* 2019;160(11): 2589–2602. doi:10.1097/j.pain.0000000000001640

34. Bazzichi L, Palego L, Giannaccini G, et al. Altered amino acid homeostasis in subjects affected by fibromyalgia. *Clin Biochem.* 2009;42(10-11):1064–1070. doi:10.1016/j.clinbiochem. 2009.02.025

35. Wu Z, Malihi Z, Stewart AW, Lawes CM, Scragg R. The association between vitamin D concentration and pain: a systematic review and meta-analysis. *Public Health Nutr.* 2018;21 (11):2022–2037. doi:10.1017/S1368980018000551

36. Cordero MD, Moreno-Fernández AM, deMiguel M, et al. Coenzyme Q10 distribution in blood is altered in patients with fibromyalgia.*Clin Biochem.* 2009;42(7-8):732–735. doi:10.1016/j. clinbiochem.2008.12.010

37. Wolfe F, Smythe HA, Yunus MB, et al. The American College of Rheumatology 1990 Criteria for the Classification of Fibromyalgia. Report of the Multicenter Criteria Committee. *Arthritis Rheum.* 1990;33(2):160–172. doi:10.1002/art. 1780330203

38. Wolfe F, Clauw DJ, Fitzcharles MA, et al. The American College of Rheumatology preliminary diagnostic criteria for fibromyalgia and measurement of symptom severity. *Arthritis Care Res (Hoboken).* 2010;62(5):600–610. doi:10.1002/acr.20140

39. Wolfe F, Clauw DJ, Fitzcharles MA, et al. 2016 Revisions to the 2010/2011 fibromyalgia diagnostic criteria. *Semin Arthritis Rheum.* 2016;46(3):319–329. doi:10.1016/j.semarthrit.2016. 08.012

40. Delves PJ. Food Allergy. Merck Manual Professional Version. https://www.merckmanuals.com/en-ca/professional/

immunology-allergic-disorders/allergic,-autoimmune,-and-other-hypersensitivity-disorders/food-allergy?query=food%20 allergy. Updated July 2019. Accessed February 5, 2020.

41. Delves PJ. Anaphylaxis. Merck Manual Professional Version. https://www.merckmanuals.com/en-ca/professional/immunology-allergic-disorders/allergic,-autoimmune,-and-other-hypersensitivity-disorders/anaphylaxis?query=anaphylaxis. Updated July 2019. Accessed February 5, 2020.

42. Rocky Mountain Analytical. IgG Food Sensitivity. https://www.rmalab.com/medical-laboratory-tests/allergy/igg-sensitivity. Accessed February 5, 2020.

43. Global Lyme Alliance. Lyme Disease Testing. https://globallymealliance.org/about-lyme/diagnosis/testing/. Accessed February 5, 2020.

44. Armin Labs. TickPlex – First Immunoassay for persister forms. https://www.arminlabs.com/en/tests/tickplex. Accessed February 5, 2020.

45. The Great Plains Laboratory, Inc. Organic Acids Test (ACT). https://www.greatplainslaboratory.com/organic-acids-test. Accessed February 5, 2020.

46. Precision Analytical Inc. DUTCH Plus. https://dutchtest.com/info-dutch-plus/. Accessed February 5, 2020.

47. Precision Analytical Inc. DUTCH Complete. https://dutchtest.com/info-dutch-complete/. Accessed February 5, 2020.

48. Riva R, Mork PJ, Westgaard RH, Rø M, Lundberg U. Fibromyalgia syndrome is associated with hypocortisolism. *Int J Behav Med.* 2010;17(3):223–233. doi:10.1007/s12529-010-9097-6

49. Izquierdo-Alvarez S, Bocos-Terraz JP, Bancalero-Flores JL, Pavón-Romero L, Serrano-Ostariz E, de Miquel CA. Is there an association between fibromyalgia and below-normal levels of urinary cortisol?. *BMC Res Notes.* 2008;1:134. Published 2008 Dec 22. doi:10.1186/1756-0500-1-134

50. Catley D, Kaell AT, Kirschbaum C, Stone AA. A naturalistic evaluation of cortisol secretion in persons with fibromyalgia and rheumatoid arthritis. *Arthritis Care Res.* 2000;13(1):51–61. doi:10.1002/1529-0131(200002)13:1<51::aid-art8>3.0.co;2-q

51. Nicolson NA, Davis MC, Kruszewski D, Zautra AJ. Childhood maltreatment and diurnal cortisol patterns in women with chronic pain. *Psychosom Med.* 2010;72(5):471–480. doi:10.1097/PSY.0b013e3181d9a104

52. Crofford LJ, Young EA, Engleberg NC, et al. Basal circadian and pulsatile ACTH and cortisol secretion in patients with fibromyalgia and/or chronic fatigue syndrome. *Brain Behav Immun.* 2004;18(4):314–325. doi:10.1016/j.bbi.2003.12.011

53. Fatima G, Das SK, Mahdi AA, et al. Circadian rhythm of serum cortisol in female patients with fibromyalgia syndrome. *Indian J Clin Biochem.* 2013;28(2):181–184. doi:10.1007/s12291-012-0258-z

54. Vakil N. *Helicobacter pylori* infection. Merck Manual Professional Version. https://www.merckmanuals.com/en-ca/professional/gastrointestinal-disorders/gastritis-and-peptic-ulcer-disease/helicobacter-pylori-infection?query=h%20pylori. Updated January 2020. Accessed February 5, 2020.

55. Doctor's Data Inc. Comprehensive Stool Analysis w/Parasitology x3. https://www.doctorsdata.com/comprehensive-stool-analysis-w-parasitology-x3/. Accessed February 5, 2020.

56. Ortancil O, Sanli A, Eryuksel R, Basaran A, Ankarali H. Association between serum ferritin level and fibromyalgia syndrome. *Eur J Clin Nutr.* 2010;64(3):308–312. doi:10.1038/ejcn.2009.149

57. Mytavin Inc. Mytavin calculate your needs. https://mytavin.com/. Accessed February 5, 2020.

58. Natural Medicines Database. Iron. https://naturalmedicines.therapeuticresearch.com/databases/food,-herbs-supplements/

professional.aspx?productid=912. Updated August 27, 2019. Accessed February 5, 2020.

59. Prousky J. *Textbook of Integrative Clinical Nutrition*. Toronto, ON: CCNM Press; 2012.

60. Regland B, Forsmark S, Halaouate L, et al. Response to vitamin B12 and folic acid in myalgic encephalomyelitis and fibromyalgia. *PLoS One*. 2015;10(4):e0124648. Published 2015 Apr 22. doi:10.1371/journal.pone.0124648

61. Natural Medicines Database. Vitamin B12. https://naturalmedicines.therapeuticresearch.com/databases/food,-herbs-supplements/professional.aspx?productid=926. Updated February 19, 2019. Accessed February 5, 2020.

62. Patel K. Vitamin D. Examine.com. https://examine.com/supplements/vitamin-d/. Updated December 30, 2019. Accessed February 5, 2020.

63. Hausteiner-Wiehle C, Henningsen P. Irritable bowel syndrome: relations with functional, mental, and somatoform disorders. *World J Gastroenterol*. 2014;20(20):6024–6030. doi:10.3748/wjg.v20.i20.6024

64. Moleski SM. Irritable Bowel Syndrome (IBS). Merck Manual Professional Version.https://www.merckmanuals.com/en-ca/professional/gastrointestinal-disorders/irritable-bowel-syndrome-ibs/irritable-bowel-syndrome-ibs?query=irritable%20bowel%20syndrome. Updated April 2019. Retrieved February 5, 2020.

65. Ghoshal UC, Shukla R, Ghoshal U. Small Intestinal Bacterial Overgrowth and Irritable Bowel Syndrome: A Bridge between Functional Organic Dichotomy. *Gut Liver*. 2017;11(2):196–208. doi:10.5009/gnl16126

66. Silberstein SD. Migraine. Merck Manual Professional Version. https://www.merckmanuals.com/en-ca/professional/neurologic-

disorders/headache/migraine?query=migraine. Updated June 2018. Accessed February 6, 2020.

67. Penn IW, Chuang E, Chuang TY, Lin CL, Kao CH. Bidirectional association between migraine and fibromyalgia: retrospective cohort analyses of two populations. *BMJ Open.* 2019;9(4):e026581. Published 2019 Apr 8. doi:10.1136/bmjopen -2018-026581

68. Alstadhaug KB, Andreou AP. Caffeine and Primary (Migraine) Headaches-Friend or Foe?. *Front Neurol.* 2019;10:1275. Published 2019 Dec 3. doi:10.3389/fneur.2019.01275

69. Schwab RJ. Periodic Limb Movement Disorder (PLMD) and Restless Legs Syndrome (RLS). Merck Manual Professional Version. https://www.merckmanuals.com/en-ca/professional/neurologic-disorders/sleep-and-wakefulness-disorders/periodic-limb-movement-disorder-plmd-and-restless-legs-syndrome-rls?query=restless%20leg%20syndrome. Updated December 2018. Accessed February 6, 2020.

70. Civelek GM, Ciftkaya PO, Karatas M. Evaluation of restless legs syndrome in fibromyalgia syndrome: an analysis of quality of sleep and life. *J Back MusculoskeletRehabil.* 2014;27(4):537–544. doi:10.3233/BMR-140478

71. Coryell W. Depressive disorders. Merck Manual Professional Version. https://www.merckmanuals.com/en-ca/professional/psychiatric-disorders/mood-disorders/depressive-disorders?query=depression. Updated May 2018. Accessed February 6, 2020.

72. Barnhill JW. Generalized anxiety disorder (GAD). Merck Manual Professional Version. https://www.merckmanuals.com/en-ca/professional/psychiatric-disorders/anxiety-and-stressor-related-disorders/generalized-anxiety-disorder-gad?query=anxiety. Updated July 2018. Accessed February 6, 2020.

73. Dukowicz AC, Lacy BE, Levine GM. Small intestinal bacterial overgrowth: a comprehensive review. *Gastroenterol Hepatol (N Y)*. 2007;3(2):112–122.

74. Pimentel M, Wallace D, Hallegua D, et al. A link between irritable bowel syndrome and fibromyalgia may be related to findings on lactulose breath testing. *Ann Rheum Dis*. 2004;63(4):450–452. doi:10.1136/ard.2003.011502

75. Gluckman S. Chronic fatigue syndrome. Merck Manual Professional Version. https://www.merckmanuals.com/en-ca/professional/special-subjects/chronic-fatigue-syndrome/chronic-fatigue-syndrome?query=chronic%20fatigue%20syndrome. Updated August 2018. Accessed February 6, 2020.

76. Black DW. Idiopathic Environmental Intolerance. Merck Manual Professional Version. https://www.merckmanuals.com/en-ca/professional/special-subjects/idiopathic-environmental-intolerance/idiopathic-environmental-intolerance?query=multiple%20chemical%20sensitivity. Updated November 2018. Accessed February 6, 2020.

77. Colten HR, Altevogt BM. *Sleep Disorders and Sleep Deprivation: An Umnet Public Health Problem*. Washington, DC: The National Academies Press; 2006. doi: 10.17226/11617. Accessed February 7, 2020.

78. Carley DW, Farabi SS. Physiology of sleep. *Diabetes Spectr*. 2016;29(1):5-9. doi:10.2337/diaspect.29.1.5.

79. Wu YL, Chang LY, Lee HC, Fang SC, Tsai PS. Sleep disturbances in fibromyalgia: A meta-analysis of case-control studies. *J Psychosom Res*. 2017;96:89–97. doi:10.1016/j.jpsychores.2017.03.011

80. Bested AC. Activity Log & Functional Capacity Scale. ME/CFS Assist. http://mecfsassist.weebly.com/activity-log--functional-capacity-scale.html. Accessed February 7, 2020.

81. Carson JW, Carson KM, Jones KD, Bennett RM, Wright CL, Mist SD. A pilot randomized controlled trial of the Yoga of

Awareness program in the management of fibromyalgia. *Pain.* 2010;151(2):530–539. doi:10.1016/j.pain.2010.08.020

82. Lazaridou A, Koulouris A, Devine JK, et al. Impact of daily yoga-based exercise on pain, catastrophizing, and sleep amongst individuals with fibromyalgia. *J Pain Res.* 2019;12:2915–2923. Published 2019 Oct 17. doi:10.2147/JPR.S210653

83. Curtis K, Osadchuk A, Katz J. An eight-week yoga intervention is associated with improvements in pain, psychological functioning and mindfulness, and changes in cortisol levels in women with fibromyalgia. *J Pain Res.* 2011;4:189–201. doi:10. 2147/JPR.S22761

84. Lazaridou A, Koulouris A, Dorado K, Chai P, Edwards RR, Schreiber KL. The Impact of a Daily Yoga Program for Women with Fibromyalgia. *Int J Yoga.* 2019;12(3):206–217. doi:10.4103/ ijoy.IJOY_72_18

85. Bidonde J, Busch AJ, Webber SC, et al. Aquatic exercise training for fibromyalgia. *Cochrane Database Syst Rev.* 2014;(10):CD011336. Published 2014 Oct 28. doi:10.1002/14651858.CD011336

86. Silva AR, Bernardo A, Costa J, et al. Dietary interventions in fibromyalgia: a systematic review. *Ann Med.* 2019;51(sup1):2–14. doi:10.1080/07853890.2018.1564360

87. Correa-Rodríguez M, Casas-Barragán A, González-Jiménez E, Schmidt-RioValle J, Molina F, Aguilar-Ferrándiz ME. Dietary Inflammatory Index Scores Are Associated with Pressure Pain Hypersensitivity in Women with Fibromyalgia [published online ahead of print, 2019 Sep 25]. *Pain Med.* 2019;pnz238. doi:10.1093/pm/pnz238

88. Marum AP, Moreira C, Saraiva F, Tomas-Carus P, Sousa-Guerreiro C. A low fermentable oligo-di-mono saccharides and polyols (FODMAP) diet reduced pain and improved daily life in fibromyalgia patients. *Scand J Pain.* 2016;13:166–172. doi:10.1016/j.sjpain.2016.07.004

89. Low FODMAP Diet. stanfordhealthcare.org. https://stanfordhealthcare.org/medical-treatments/l/low-fodmap-diet.html. Accessed February 7, 2020.

90. Murray MT, Pizzorno J. *The Encyclopedia of Natural Medicine.* 3rd ed. New York, NY: Atria Paperback; 2012.

91. Frequently Asked Questions about Pesticides and Produce. ewg.org. https://www.ewg.org/foodnews/faq.php. Accessed February 7, 2020.

92. Shoppers Guide to Pesticides in Produce. ewg.org. https://www.ewg.org/foodnews/. Accessed February 7, 2020.

93. Consumer Guides. ewg.org. https://www.ewg.org/consumer-guides. Accessed February 7, 2020.

94. Andrés-Rodríguez L, Borràs X, Feliu-Soler A, et al. Immune-inflammatory pathways and clinical changes in fibromyalgia patients treated with Mindfulness-Based Stress Reduction (MBSR): A randomized, controlled clinical trial. *Brain Behav Immun.* 2019;80:109–119. doi:10.1016/j.bbi.2019.02.030

95. Lauche R, Cramer H, Dobos G, Langhorst J, Schmidt S. A systematic review and meta-analysis of mindfulness-based stress reduction for the fibromyalgia syndrome. *J Psychosom Res.* 2013;75(6):500–510. doi:10.1016/j.jpsychores.2013.10.010

96. Haugmark T, Hagen KB, Smedslund G, Zangi HA. Mindfulness- and acceptance-based interventions for patients with fibromyalgia - A systematic review and meta-analyses. *PLoS One.* 2019;14(9):e0221897. Published 2019 Sep 3. doi:10.1371/journal.pone.0221897

97. EWG's Tap Water Database. ewg.org. https://www.ewg.org/tapwater/. Accessed February 8, 2020.

98. Water Talk – Lead in Drinking Water. canada.ca. https://www.canada.ca/en/health-canada/services/environmental-workplace-health/reports-publications/water-quality/water-

talk-minimizing-exposure-lead-drinking-water-distribution-systems.html. Accessed February 8, 2020.

99. The Dirty Secret of Government Drinking Water Standards. ewg.org. https://www.ewg.org/tapwater/state-of-american-drinking-water.php. Accessed February 8, 2020.

100. EWG's Water Filter Guide. Ewg.org. https://www.ewg.org/tapwater/water-filter-guide.php. Accessed February 8, 2020.

101. McCrindle LS, Bested AC. *The Complete Fibromyalgia Health, Diet Guide & Cookbook: Includes Practical Wellness Solutions & 100 Delicious Recipes*. Toronto, ON: Robert Rose Inc.; 2013.

102. Mytavin [Calculate Your Needs]. mytavin.com. https://mytavin.com/. Accessed February 8, 2020.

103. Gropper SS, Smith JL, Groff JL. *Advanced Nutrition and Human Metabolism*. 5th ed. Belmont, CA: Wadsworth; 2009.

104. Thiamin. naturalmedicines.therapeuticresearch.com. https://naturalmedicines.therapeuticresearch.com/databases/food,-herbs-supplements/professional.aspx?productid=965. Accessed February 8, 2020.

105. Riboflacin. naturalmedicines.therapeuticresearch.com. https://naturalmedicines.therapeuticresearch.com/databases/food,-herbs-supplements/professional.aspx?productid=957. Accessed February 8, 2020.

106. Niacin. naturalmedicines.therapeuticresearch.com. https://naturalmedicines.therapeuticresearch.com/databases/food,-herbs-supplements/professional.aspx?productid=924. Accessed February 8, 2020.

107. Pantothenic Acid. naturalmedicines.therapeuticresearch.com. https://naturalmedicines.therapeuticresearch.com/databases/food,-herbs-supplements/professional.aspx?productid=853. Accessed February 8, 2020.

108. Biotin. naturalmedicines.therapeuticresearch.com. https://naturalmedicines.therapeuticresearch.com/databases/food,-

herbs-supplements/professional.aspx?productid=313. Accessed
February 8, 2020.

109. Folic Acid. naturalmedicines.therapeuticresearch.com. https://
naturalmedicines.therapeuticresearch.com/databases/food,-
herbs-supplements/professional.aspx?productid=1017. Accessed
February 8, 2020.

110. Vitamin B6. naturalmedicines.therapeuticresearch.com. https://
naturalmedicines.therapeuticresearch.com/databases/food,-
herbs-supplements/professional.aspx?productid=934. Accessed
February 8, 2020.

111. Patel, K. Magnesium. examine.com. https://examine.com/
supplements/magnesium/. Accessed February 8, 2020.

112. Wax W. Magnesium in diet. medlineplus.gov. https://medlineplus.
gov/ency/article/002423.htm. Accessed February 8, 2020.

113. Glycine. naturalmedicines.therapeuticresearch.com. https://
naturalmedicines.therapeuticresearch.com/databases/food,-
herbs-supplements/professional.aspx?productid=1072. Accessed
February 8, 2020.

114. Russell IJ, Michalek JE, Flechas JD, Abraham GE. Treatment of
fibromyalgia syndrome with Super Malic: a randomized, double
blind, placebo controlled, crossover pilot study. *J Rheumatol.*
1995;22(5):953–958.

115. Patel K. Iron. examine.com. https://examine.com/supplements/
iron/. Accessed February 8, 2020.

116. Geerligs PD, Brabin BJ, Omari AA. Food prepared in iron
cooking pots as an intervention for reducing iron deficiency
anaemia in developing countries: a systematic review. *J Hum Nutr
Diet.* 2003;16(4):275–281. doi:10.1046/j.1365-277x.2003.00447.x

117. Glycine. naturalmedicines.therapeuticresearch.com. https://
naturalmedicines.therapeuticresearch.com/databases/food,-
herbs-supplements/professional.aspx?productid=912. Accessed
February 8, 2020.

118. Patel K. Vitamin D. examine.com. https://examine.com/supplements/vitamin-d/. Accessed February 8, 2020.

119. Vitamin D Deficiency. my.cleavelandclinic.org. https://my.clevelandclinic.org/health/articles/15050-vitamin-d--vitamin-d-deficiency. Updated October 16, 2019. Accessed February 8, 2020.

120. Martins YA, Cardinali CAEF, Ravanelli MI, Brunaldi K. Is hypovitaminosis D associated with fibromyalgia? A systematic review. *Nutr Rev.* 2020;78(2):115–133. doi:10.1093/nutrit/nuz033

121. Karras S, Rapti E, Matsoukas S, Kotsa K. Vitamin D in Fibromyalgia: A Causative or Confounding Biological Interplay?. *Nutrients.* 2016;8(6):343. Published 2016 Jun 4. doi:10.3390/nu8060343

122. Melatonin. naturalmedicines.therapeuticresearch.com. https://naturalmedicines.therapeuticresearch.com/databases/food,-herbs-supplements/professional.aspx?productid=940. Accessed February 8, 2020.

123. Theanine. naturalmedicines.therapeuticresearch.com. https://naturalmedicines.therapeuticresearch.com/databases/food,-herbs-supplements/professional.aspx?productid=1053. Accessed February 8, 2020.

124. 5-HTP. naturalmedicines.therapeuticresearch.com. https://naturalmedicines.therapeuticresearch.com/databases/food,-herbs-supplements/professional.aspx?productid=794. Accessed February 8, 2020.

125. Magnesium. naturalmedicines.therapeuticresearch.com. https://naturalmedicines.therapeuticresearch.com/databases/food,-herbs-supplements/professional.aspx?productid=998. Accessed February 8, 2020.

126. Passion Flower. naturalmedicines.therapeuticresearch.com. https://naturalmedicines.therapeuticresearch.com/databases/

food,-herbs-supplements/professional.aspx?productid=871. Accessed February 8, 2020.

127. Valerian. naturalmedicines.therapeuticresearch.com. https:// naturalmedicines.therapeuticresearch.com/databases/food,- herbs-supplements/professional.aspx?productid=870. Accessed February 8, 2020.

128. Gas: Fun Facts about Farting and Burping. health.clevelandclinic. org. https://health.clevelandclinic.org/gas-fun-facts-flatulence- burping-infographic/. Accessed February 8, 2020.

129. Hoffman D. *Medical Herbalism: The Science and Practice of Herbal Medicine.* Rochester, VT: Healing Arts Press; 2003.

130. Gentian. naturalmedicines.therapeuticresearch.com. https:// naturalmedicines.therapeuticresearch.com/databases/food,- herbs-supplements/professional.aspx?productid=716. Accessed February 8, 2020.

131. Angelica. naturalmedicines.therapeuticresearch.com. https:// naturalmedicines.therapeuticresearch.com/databases/food,- herbs-supplements/professional.aspx?productid=281. Accessed February 8, 2020.

132. Pimpinella. naturalmedicines.therapeuticresearch.com. https:// naturalmedicines.therapeuticresearch.com/databases/food,- herbs-supplements/professional.aspx?productid=219. Accessed February 8, 2020.

133. Damiana. naturalmedicines.therapeuticresearch.com. https:// naturalmedicines.therapeuticresearch.com/databases/food,- herbs-supplements/professional.aspx?productid=703. Accessed February 8, 2020.

134. Lactobacillus. naturalmedicines.therapeuticresearch.com. https://naturalmedicines.therapeuticresearch.com/databases/ food,-herbs-supplements/professional.aspx?productid=790. Accessed February 8, 2020.

135. Bifidobacteria. naturalmedicines.therapeuticresearch.com. https://naturalmedicines.therapeuticresearch.com/databases/food,-herbs-supplements/professional.aspx?productid=891. Accessed February 8, 2020.

136. Glutamine. naturalmedicines.therapeuticresearch.com. https://naturalmedicines.therapeuticresearch.com/databases/food,-herbs-supplements/professional.aspx?productid=878. Accessed February 8, 2020.

137. Coenzyme Q10. naturalmedicines.therapeuticresearch.com. https://naturalmedicines.therapeuticresearch.com/databases/food,-herbs-supplements/professional.aspx?productid=938. Accessed February 8, 2020.

138. Carpenter K, Barigent MJ. Vitamin-like substances. britannica.com. https://www.britannica.com/science/vitamin/Vitamin-like-substances. Published June 14, 2019. Accessed February 8, 2020.

139. Di Pierro F, Rossi A, Consensi A, Giacomelli C, Bazzichi L. Role for a water-soluble form of CoQ10 in female subjects affected by fibromyalgia. A preliminary study. *Clin Exp Rheumatol.* 2017;35 Suppl 105(3):20–27.

140. Cordero MD, Alcocer-Gómez E, de Miguel M, et al. Can coenzyme q10 improve clinical and molecular parameters in fibromyalgia?. *Antioxid Redox Signal.* 2013;19(12):1356–1361. doi:10.1089/ars.2013.5260

141. Cordero MD, Santos-García R, Bermejo-Jover D, Sánchez-Domínguez B, Jaramillo-Santos MR, Bullón P. Coenzyme Q10 in salivary cells correlate with blood cells in Fibromyalgia: improvement in clinical and biochemical parameter after oral treatment. *Clin Biochem.* 2012;45(6):509–511. doi:10.1016/j.clinbiochem.2012.02.001

142. Cordero MD, Cano-García FJ, Alcocer-Gómez E, De Miguel M, Sánchez-Alcázar JA. Oxidative stress correlates with headache symptoms in fibromyalgia: coenzyme $Q_{10}$ effect on clinical

improvement. *PLoS One*. 2012;7(4):e35677. doi:10.1371/journal. pone.0035677

143. Low blood pressure (hypotension). mayoclinic.org. https:// www.mayoclinic.org/diseases-conditions/low-blood-pressure/ symptoms-causes/syc-20355465. Updated March 10, 2018. Accessed February 8, 2020.

144. Acetyl-L-Carnitine. naturalmedicines.therapeuticresearch.com. https://naturalmedicines.therapeuticresearch.com/databases/ food,-herbs-supplements/professional.aspx?productid=834. Accessed February 8, 2020.

145. Rossini M, Di Munno O, Valentini G, et al. Double-blind, multicenter trial comparing acetyl l-carnitine with placebo in the treatment of fibromyalgia patients. *Clin Exp Rheumatol*. 2007;25(2):182–188.

146. Leombruni P, Miniotti M, Colonna F, et al. A randomised controlled trial comparing duloxetine and acetyl L-carnitine in fibromyalgic patients: preliminary data. *Clin Exp Rheumatol*. 2015;33(1 Suppl 88):S82–S85.

147. Alpha-Lipoic Acid. naturalmedicines.therapeuticresearch.com. https://naturalmedicines.therapeuticresearch.com/databases/ food,-herbs-supplements/professional.aspx?productid=767. Accessed February 8, 2020.

148. Gilron I, Tu D, Holden R, Towheed T, Vandenkerkhof E, Milev R. Combination Analgesic Development for Enhanced Clinical Efficacy (CADENCE Trial): Study Protocol for a Double-Blind, Randomized, Placebo-Controlled Crossover Trial of an Alpha-Lipoic Acid - Pregabalin Combination for the Treatment of Fibromyalgia Pain. *JMIR Res Protoc*. 2017;6(8):e154. Published 2017 Aug 4. doi:10.2196/resprot.8001

149. Gilron I, Tu D, Holden R, et al. Innovations in the Management of Musculoskeletal Pain With Alpha-Lipoic Acid (IMPALA Trial): Study protocol for a Double-Blind, Randomized,

Placebo-Controlled Crossover Trial of Alpha-Lipoic Acid for the Treatment of Fibromyalgia Pain. *JMIR Res Protoc.* 2017;6(3):e41. Published 2017 Mar 28. doi:10.2196/resprot.7198

150. Ribose. naturalmedicines.therapeuticresearch.com. https:// naturalmedicines.therapeuticresearch.com/databases/food,- herbs-supplements/professional.aspx?productid=827. Accessed February 8, 2020.

151. Teitelbaum JE, Johnson C, St Cyr J. The use of D-ribose in chronic fatigue syndrome and fibromyalgia: a pilot study. *J Altern Complement Med.* 2006;12(9):857–862. doi:10.1089/ acm.2006.12.857

152. Gebhart B, Jorgenson JA. Benefit of ribose in a patient with fibromyalgia. *Pharmacotherapy.* 2004;24(11):1646–1648. doi:10.1592/phco.24.16.1646.50957

153. Palmitoylethanolamide (PEA). naturalmedicines.therapeutic research.com. https://naturalmedicines.therapeuticresearch. com/databases/food,-herbs-supplements/professional.aspx? productid=1596. Accessed February 10, 2020.

154. Skaper SD, Facci L, Zusso M, Giusti P. An Inflammation-Centric View of Neurological Disease: Beyond the Neuron. *Front Cell Neurosci.* 2018;12:72. Published 2018 Mar 21. doi:10.3389/ fncel.2018.00072

155. Paladini A, Fusco M, Cenacchi T, Schievano C, Piroli A, Varrassi G. Palmitoylethanolamide, a Special Food for Medical Purposes, in the Treatment of Chronic Pain: A Pooled Data Meta-analysis. *Pain Physician.* 2016;19(2):11–24.

156. Artukoglu BB, Beyer C, Zuloff-Shani A, Brener E, Bloch MH. Efficacy of Palmitoylethanolamide for Pain: A Meta-Analysis. *Pain Physician.* 2017;20(5):353–362.

157. Schweiger V, Martini A, Bellamoli P, et al. Ultramicronized Palmitoylethanolamide (um-PEA) as Add-on Treatment in Fibromyalgia Syndrome (FMS): Retrospective Observational

Study on 407 Patients. *CNS Neurol Disord Drug Targets.* 2019;18(4):326–333. doi:10.2174/1871527318666190227205359

158. Del Giorno R, Skaper S, Paladini A, Varrassi G, Coaccioli S. Palmitoylethanolamide in Fibromyalgia: Results from Prospective and Retrospective Observational Studies. *Pain Ther.* 2015;4(2):169–178. doi:10.1007/s40122-015-0038-6

159. Turmeric. naturalmedicines.therapeuticresearch.com. https:// naturalmedicines.therapeuticresearch.com/databases/food,- herbs-supplements/professional.aspx?productid=662. Accessed February 10, 2020.

160. Langhorst J, Musial F, Klose P, Häuser W. Efficacy of hydrotherapy in fibromyalgia syndrome--a meta-analysis of randomized controlled clinical trials. *Rheumatology (Oxford).* 2009;48(9):1155–1159. doi:10.1093/rheumatology/kep182

161. McVeigh JG, McGaughey H, Hall M, Kane P. The effectiveness of hydrotherapy in the management of fibromyalgia syndrome: a systematic review. *Rheumatol Int.* 2008;29(2):119–130. doi:10. 1007/s00296-008-0674-9

162. Boswellia. naturalmedicines.therapeuticresearch.com. https:// naturalmedicines.therapeuticresearch.com/databases/food,- herbs-supplements/professional.aspx?productid=63. Accessed February 10, 2020.

163. Devil's Claw. naturalmedicines.therapeuticresearch.com. https:// naturalmedicines.therapeuticresearch.com/databases/food,- herbs-supplements/professional.aspx?productid=984. Accessed February 10, 2020.

164. Murray MT, Pizzorno J. *The Encyclopedia of Natural Medicine.* 3rd ed. New York, NY: Atria Paperback; 2012.

165. Winston D, Maimes S. *Adaptogens: Herbs for Strength, Stamina, and Stress Relief.* Rochester, YT: Healing Arts Press; 2007.

166. Holy Basil. naturalmedicines.therapeuticresearch.com. https:// naturalmedicines.therapeuticresearch.com/databases/food,-

herbs-supplements/professional.aspx?productid=1101. Accessed February 10, 2020.

167. Rhodiola. naturalmedicines.therapeuticresearch.com. https:// naturalmedicines.therapeuticresearch.com/databases/food,- herbs-supplements/professional.aspx?productid=883. Accessed February 10, 2020.

168. Ashwagandha. naturalmedicines.therapeuticresearch.com. https://naturalmedicines.therapeuticresearch.com/databases/ food,-herbs-supplements/professional.aspx?productid=953. Accessed February 10, 2020.

169. Licorice. naturalmedicines.therapeuticresearch.com. https:// naturalmedicines.therapeuticresearch.com/databases/food,- herbs-supplements/professional.aspx?productid=881. Accessed February 10, 2020.

170. Panax Ginseng. naturalmedicines.therapeuticresearch.com. https://naturalmedicines.therapeuticresearch.com/databases/ food,-herbs-supplements/professional.aspx?productid=1000. Accessed February 10, 2020.

171. Braz AS, Morais LC, Paula AP, Diniz MF, Almeida RN. Effects of Panax ginseng extract in patients with fibromyalgia: a 12-week, randomized, double-blind, placebo-controlled trial. *Braz J Psychiatry*. 2013;35(1):21–28. doi:10.1016/j.rbp.2013.01.004

172. Eleuthero. naturalmedicines.therapeuticresearch.com. https:// naturalmedicines.therapeuticresearch.com/databases/food,- herbs-supplements/professional.aspx?productid=985. Accessed February 10, 2020.

173. Løge-Hagen JS, Sæle A, Juhl C, Bech P, Stenager E, Mellentin AI. Prevalence of depressive disorder among patients with fibromyalgia: Systematic review and meta-analysis. *J Affect Disord*. 2019;245:1098–1105. doi:10.1016/j.jad.2018.12.001

174. Bondesson E, Larrosa Pardo F, Stigmar K, et al. Comorbidity between pain and mental illness - Evidence of a bidirectional

relationship. *Eur J Pain*. 2018;22(7):1304–1311. doi:10.1002/ejp.1218

175. Gamma-Aminobutyric Acid (GABA). naturalmedicines.therapeuticresearch.com. https://naturalmedicines.therapeuticresearch.com/databases/food,-herbs-supplements/professional.aspx?productid=464. Accessed February 10, 2020.

176. Caruso I, SarziPuttini P, Cazzola M, Azzolini V. Double-blind study of 5-hydroxytryptophan versus placebo in the treatment of primary fibromyalgia syndrome. *J Int Med Res*. 1990;18(3):201–209. doi:10.1177/030006059001800304

177. SarziPuttini P, Caruso I. Primary fibromyalgia syndrome and 5-hydroxy-L-tryptophan: a 90-day open study. *J Int Med Res*. 1992;20(2):182–189. doi:10.1177/030006059202000210

178. SAMe. naturalmedicines.therapeuticresearch.com. https://naturalmedicines.therapeuticresearch.com/databases/food,-herbs-supplements/professional.aspx?productid=786. Accessed February 10, 2020.

179. Jacobsen S, Danneskiold-Samsøe B, Andersen RB. Oral S-adenosylmethionine in primary fibromyalgia. Double-blind clinical evaluation. *Scand J Rheumatol*. 1991;20(4):294–302. doi:10.3109/03009749109096803

180. What You Need To Know About Iron. UnlockFood.ca. https://www.unlockfood.ca/en/Articles/Vitamins-and-Minerals/What-You-Need-To-Know-About-Iron.aspx. Updated February 14, 2019. Accessed February 12, 2020.

181. How To Get More Iron. UnlckFood.ca. https://www.unlockfood.ca/en/Articles/Vitamins-and-Minerals/How-To-Get-More-Iron.aspx#.VuCfuJMrKRs. Updated September 8, 2019. Accessed February 12, 2020.

# ACKNOWLEDGMENTS

Thank you to all of my patients who trust me with a part their health journey. I am honoured to be a part of it and proud of how much each and every one of you have achieved and continue to achieve.

Thanks to the readers of this book. You inspire me to continue to work towards improving the health care available to those with fibromyalgia.

A big thank you to my dear friend Michelle Mussar. You have been a constant source of encouragement and excitement since before this book had a home on paper. This book truly would not be in existence if it weren't for you!

I owe a world of gratitude to my mom, Cindy, and my aunts, Lynda and Karen, who assisted me with the big goal of becoming a naturopathic doctor. None of this would not have been possible without your support.

Thanks to my mom, Dave, Sarah, Emily, Donna, Gino, Alanna, and Luis for your encouragement and support. You've been cheering me on at every step of the way and I appreciate it more than I could ever express.

And finally, a big thank you to my partner, Daniel, for your patience and care while I turned my dream into a reality. Your constant reminders to take a break, go to sleep, and eat something did not go unnoticed or unappreciated.

# ABOUT THE AUTHOR

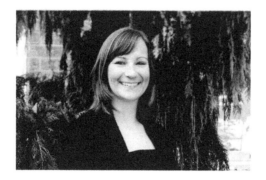

Melyssa Hoitink is a naturopathic doctor with a practice focused on treating fibromyalgia in Barrie, Ontario. Prior to becoming a naturopathic doctor, Melyssa completed a Bachelor of Science degree, majoring in Human Nutritional Sciences at the University of Manitoba in Winnipeg, Manitoba. She then went on to complete her Doctor of Naturopathy degree at the Canadian College of Naturopathic Medicine. During her training, she completed a 12-month focused internship in caring for patients with fibromyalgia and myalgic encephalomyelitis (also known as chronic fatigue syndrome), which sparked her passion for working with this enthusiastic population.

In her free time, Melyssa can be found outdoors on the water with a book in hand. She enjoys spending time with her family, friends, and her partner, Daniel. Melyssa lives in Innisfil, Ontario with Daniel and their fur babies.

Visit Melyssa's website at: www.drmelyssa.com
Instagram and Facebook: @drmelyssa.nd

# Can You Help?

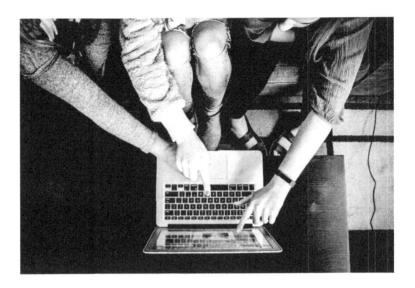

## Thank You for Reading My Book!

I really appreciate all of your feedback, and
I love hearing what you have to say.

I need your input to make the next version of
this book and my future books better.

Please leave me an honest review on Amazon
letting me know what you thought of the book.

Thanks so much!

Dr. Melyssa

Made in the USA
Coppell, TX
20 February 2024

29207698R00164